Management of Distressing Bodily Symptoms in Health

I0093503

Somatisation or medically unexplained symptoms (MUS) are distressing bodily symptoms for which tests and scans return normal. They can be incredibly debilitating conditions and people seek health care frequently due to their distress. They are common worldwide – yet there are few interventions available to help those suffering with the physical and emotional pain they cause. This book presents a solution to this problem by providing a comprehensive introduction to The BodyMind Approach (TBMA), developed by Helen Payne, and outlines guidance on applying TBMA principles to facilitated groupwork with patients/clients.

Readers will learn how TBMA's biopsychosocial learning model can be used to support patients in their self-management of anxiety associated with body distress disorder, as well as their accompanying bodily felt experience.

Chapters explore:

- Adult learning theories and The BodyMind Approach
- An overview of medically unexplained symptoms/body distress disorder
- The BodyMind Approach
- The BodyMind Approach Programme
- Training of The BodyMind Approach facilitators
- Qualitative research on The BodyMind Approach
- Somatisation and adult attachment theory
- The BodyMind Approach to support students in higher education
- Somatisation, The BodyMind Approach and chronic stress

This unique book is essential reading for healthcare professionals and mental health practitioners, as well as those who are, or wish to train, as a TBMA facilitator. It will also be a compelling read for a variety of other professions, including, but not limited to, dance movement psychotherapists, art psychotherapists, counsellors, health coaches, clinical psychologists, GPs, pain clinic staff and nurses.

Helen Payne, PhD, Professor of Psychotherapy, has been researching somatic symptoms since 2005. She works part time at the University of Hertfordshire conducting research and supervising doctoral students in the School of Life and Medical Sciences, department of Psychology. In 2012 she led the formation of Pathways2Wellbeing as Director and Clinical Manager for delivering TBMA in primary healthcare. She is a trainer in the Discipline of Authentic Movement.

Susan Brooks, MSc, MA, MSc, MBA, has worked as a teacher, social worker, biologist, senior manager, assistant chief probation officer and university senior lecturer. Susan offers an unusual skill mix which brings a holistic and truly biopsychosocial perspective to the understanding of distressing bodily symptoms. She joined Helen in 2012 as a Director in forming and managing the University of Hertfordshire spin out Pathways2Wellbeing and collaborated on the research projects.

Management of Distressing Bodily Symptoms in Health

The BodyMind Approach: Using a Biopsychosocial Model

Helen Payne and Susan Brooks

Routledge
Taylor & Francis Group

LONDON AND NEW YORK

First published 2025
by Routledge
4 Park Square, Milton Park, Abingdon, Oxon OX14 4RN

and by Routledge
605 Third Avenue, New York, NY 10158

Routledge is an imprint of the Taylor & Francis Group, an informa business

British Library Cataloguing-in-Publication Data
A catalogue record for this book is available from the British Library

ISBN: 978-1-032-60845-7 (hbk)
ISBN: 978-1-032-60843-3 (pbk)
ISBN: 978-1-003-46074-9 (ebk)

DOI: 10.4324/9781003460749

Typeset in Sabon
by Newgen Publishing UK

To all the patient-participants, facilitators and trainers
who have engaged with the delivery and training in
The BodyMind Approach.

Contents

List of Figures and Tables

Figures

Tables

Disclaimer

The interventions and materials in this book may be beyond the authorised practice of mental health professionals. As a licensed professional you are responsible for reviewing the scope of practice including activities defined in law as beyond the boundaries of practice in accordance and compliance with your profession's standards. It is recommended that full TBMA facilitator training is undertaken before delivering the practices to clients/patients.

Acknowledgements

The authors would like to thank the University of Hertfordshire for their support in the development of The BodyMind Approach for patients with medically unexplained symptoms. Much appreciation goes to Silvana Reynolds for her long-standing contribution as a facilitator, and now trainer in TBMA. We also appreciate the publisher, Routledge, for their help in shaping the content of the book and Redouane Ibrahim and Jane Batchelor for their efforts assisting us on producing this book in their role as student research assistants. Finally, Helen would like to send appreciations to her family for their patience and support in her endeavours.

Preface

Undiagnosed distressing, chronic, physical symptoms where no organic cause has been found have been termed medically unexplained symptoms (MUS) in the past. In this book we have employed the term `somatisation' and used this interchangeably with the terms MUS and body distress disorder (BDD) (the most recent umbrella term for these symptoms and for diagnosed conditions both often accompanied by significant anxiety and/or depression). Medically unexplained symptoms can be incredibly debilitating conditions and people seek health care frequently due to their distress. They are common worldwide – yet there are few interventions available to help those suffering with the physical and emotional pain they cause. This book presents a solution to this problem by providing a comprehensive introduction to The BodyMind Approach (TBMA), developed by Helen Payne, and outlines guidance on applying TBMA principles to facilitated groupwork with patients/clients. Somatisation is generally defined as the tendency to experience psychological distress in the form of somatic symptoms and seek medical help. In this term includes physical symptoms for which tests and scans come back as normal and the emotional distress associated with these symptoms.

The following questions are explored:

How can working with the body help people with chronic bodily symptoms for which all tests come back normal?

How can working with the interrelationship of body and mind develop greater self-management?

How can we help health professionals to work more effectively with chronic bodily symptoms for which there is excessive emotional distress?

This book holds some of the answers.

The aim is to showcase entirely new material developed specifically for this book as well as a few published, yet updated, articles on novel intervention called The BodyMind Approach, researched at the University of Hertfordshire, and delivered with encouraging outcomes in the NHS. The book aims to enlighten health professionals, patients and trainees in The BodyMind Approach.

The book shares insights into the delivery of TBMA which has been designed as a self-management intervention for patients with chronic bodily symptoms for which all tests and scans return negative. The scope of the book covers the subjects of medically unexplained symptoms now included in the term body distress disorder, therefore the authors have named them both as somatisation. The book describes the aetiology of MUS and BDD; how TBMA is designed as a perceptual learning approach; TBMA programme; the facilitator training; qualitative research into TBMA; the link between insecure attachment and MUS; stress in higher education students and MUS; and the stress response in MUS. Finally, there is an epilogue which looks towards the future.

Introduction

Background

This chapter invites the reader to delve into the background of medically unexplained symptoms/body distress disorder and The BodyMind Approach (TBMA). Somatisation in this book is defined as the tendency to experience emotional distress in the form of, and due to, chronic somatic symptoms and to perpetually seek medical help for them. These symptoms may be initiated and/or prolonged by emotional responses such as stress, anxiety and/or depression. This book delves deeply into the biopsychosocial approach within the context of embodied perceptual learning. The aim of the intervention described in this book called TBMA is to support self-management for people experiencing persistent and chronic somatisation, whether medically explained symptoms (MUS) or those explained with an organic diagnosis. This change to encompass an organic diagnosis when accompanied by disproportionate stress/anxiety is a relatively recent one. There is another term used, health anxiety, which is a fear and preoccupation with the belief that one has, or is in danger of developing, a serious illness like cancer or a heart attack. This belief takes over one's life. There is a drive by both doctors and patients to give a name to any condition, which is understandable. Doctors are driven to find a diagnosis for their patient as this enables them to decide on the course of treatment and patients also feel reassured by a diagnosis. Where there is no organic diagnosis, the name given to patients is a label such as fibromyalgia, irritable bowel syndrome (IBS), chronic pain and/or fatigue and so on. Alternatively, since all tests and scans return normal, there is no label or diagnosis, hence in the past the term used was MUS, although it was rarely offered to the patient, who was told instead simply that there was nothing amiss (albeit the patient still experiences the body distress).

Historically there has been a dualism between physical and mental health. However, physical/organic categories overlap with psychological/mental categories in a third category which interfaces between them. There is still stigma attached to mental health conditions, so it is important to recognise this interface whereby both categories are important for diagnosis and treatment.

DOI: 10.4324/9781003460749-1

Creed et al. (2010) found the term MUS unacceptable to patients and less holistic; this has resulted in a new diagnosis for both MUS and symptoms with a physical explanation of body distress disorder (BDD) as a third category. There have been many terms to describe these conditions (please see the Appendix for a list of synonyms) each of which has attempted to better describe the condition for doctors and patients. Since there is such a proliferation of terms the authors of this book have decided to use the term somatisation, as an umbrella term to cover both MUS and BDD and any synonyms for these conditions. At times readers will see the term MUS or MUS/BDD or indeed somatisation.

Medically Unexplained Symptoms/Body Distress Disorder

Most of the research to date has been on MUS and hence for simplicity we have continued to use the term in places in this book. However, there is a move to describe the MUS condition as BDD which removes the requirement that it is unexplained, but as yet, there is little research using this term. Both medically explained and unexplained symptoms are included in BDD. One important key feature in the diagnosis of BDD is that the notion of the patient not being believed disappears, as they are seen to have excessive emotional distress whether or not the symptoms are organic in origin. It is the degree to which the patient expresses anxiety about their symptoms which is the deciding factor.

Body Distress Disorder is a diagnosis for an individual who experiences too much distress due to a persistent or recurrent (e.g., chronic pain, fatigue) bodily symptom or symptoms, to the degree that there is a distress, attention on and preoccupation with the symptom(s) that interfere with daily functioning. The term BDD replaces the old category of MUS used in International Classification of Diseases (ICD)-10. In the DSM5 the concept of somatoform disorders has been replaced by "Somatic Symptom Disorder". A change in the new criteria is that BDD can exist with any somatic/physical illness. The bodily distress does not have to be unexplained medically.

The authors have wrestled with the implications of the change in terminology from MUS to BDD in DSM5 and ICD-11. These include: a) the fact that in BDD the organic diagnosis may be known, and b) BDD can encompass psychological issues such as anxiety/depression as mental health concerns. This has made the authors consider the relevance of TBMA to diagnosed medical conditions/mental health conditions, because TBMA is a programme based on perceptual learning rather than a psychological treatment, albeit trauma informed. However, many elements of The BodyMind Approach programme lend themselves to modifying the stress responses to bodily sensations and associated anxiety and depression. In the research, participants expressed relief from the distressing symptoms, anxiety and/or depression and increased wellbeing and activity levels linking these improvements to the facilitated

TBMA group experience (Payne & Brooks, 2016). The authors have therefore concluded that there is a strong likelihood TBMA may be relevant to BDD. In this book the authors have selected places where it is relevant in addition to MUS to include BDD, showing it as MUS/BDD or somatisation.

In our view in BDD, the associated somatic symptoms – such as headache, back ache or IBS – which are unconnected to the physical diagnosed condition (medically explained) are most likely the result of excessive anxiety about that diagnosed condition. It may be that these symptoms can be worked with via TBMA as well as the excessive anxiety which is usually present.

The condition termed MUS is now included in the term BDD which refers to there being an outcome of excessive body distress rather than the descriptive model of MUS. Furthermore, BDD labels the symptoms as a disorder rather than implying there is nothing medically wrong, even though the organic cause may still be unknown. It is characterised by chronic persistent somatic symptoms that bring excessive and disproportionate thoughts, feelings and behaviours regarding those symptoms and/or are very distressing or result in significant disruption of functioning. To be diagnosed with BDD, the individual must be persistently symptomatic for at least six months. The American Psychological Association's Diagnostic and Statistical Manual of Mental Disorders (DSM5) (APA, 2013) made significant changes to the criteria and removed the overlap across the somatoform disorders and clarified their boundaries. These changes are said to better reflect the complex interface between mental and physical health.

Another key change in the DSM5 criteria is that while MUS/BDD were a key feature for many of the disorders in DSM5, a BDD diagnosis does not require that the somatic symptoms are medically unexplained. In other words, symptoms and/or co-morbid anxiety may or may not be associated with a diagnosed medical condition. Nevertheless, at the time of TBMA research, referrals were concerned solely with patients whose tests and scans all returned as normal. Unless Western society changes its views on mental and physical health to become holistic, combining mental and physical health as one, symptoms with no organic pathology will remain unexplained.

The previously published articles in this book which referred to MUS solely have not been fully amended to reflect this change in terminology. It is important that patients have an acceptable term for their condition and have a service relevant for that condition, especially when so many refuse mental health services and pain clinics, often these are either irrelevant or do not help.

Where we have explored MUS, our working definition is as follows: "A clinical and social predicament, which includes a broad spectrum of presentations where there is difficulty accounting for symptoms based on known pathology" (Edwards et al. 2010, p. 209). This definition avoids the challenge of choosing either an organic or a psychological explanation enabling a biopsychosocial treatment to address both hypotheses. Labels for these functional somatic symptoms include fibromyalgia, non-cardiac chest pain, headache, backache and IBS.

These changes are just as much political as medical enabling clinical psychologists to recommend CBT to patients for the anxiety/depression co-morbid with the bodily symptoms. However, this omits the bodily distress element entirely. Both need to be worked with together as in TBMA.

The diagnosis can be given more easily where there are also coexisting medical problems. It avoids the tendency to conclude there is no condition. Interestingly, ICD-11 still has separate chapters for mental and physical conditions, again reflecting the dichotomous structure of the medical system. In the new DSM6, expected in 2025, the term MUS/BDD may change again.

The BodyMind Approach: Origins and Development

This next section illustrates the two authors' backgrounds and contributions to the development of The BodyMind Approach (TBMA). TBMA was originally designed for people experiencing physical (somatic) symptoms which do not appear to have an organic cause and remain medically unexplained despite tests and scans, previously termed MUS.

The first author, Helen, was invited in 2001, to consider her next topic for research at the university. On searching the literature for something which linked to her research interest in dance movement psychotherapy (DMP) she came across the term "psychosomatic" in health psychology. On searching further into this topic, it appeared to be ideal for DMP research since it spoke to both psyche and soma. This resonance between mind and body flagged up the patient population who experienced bodily symptoms which had no medical explanation. Firstly, there did not appear to be any treatment or cure for such symptoms. Secondly, they were often referred for mental health treatment which was unsuccessful or which they withdrew from in large numbers. Pain clinics were the other option for patients in pain, which were often reported as not appearing to help either. Medications from GPs were mostly anti-depressants, which seemed to reduce some symptoms, e.g., chronic pain. Overall, there were no effective treatments and those that were in place divided the person into either physical or mental health. Since Helen viewed DMP to be an intervention capable of addressing both physical and emotional needs, it occurred to her that she could perhaps explore how DMP might be helpful, or not, to this patient population (see Payne, 2025 for further description of adapted Authentic Movement /AM). A pilot study was then implemented (Payne, 2009a, 2009b, 2009c). In each of these aforementioned articles the evolution of TBMA is illustrated. For example, although the intervention started as DMP, it then morphed into DMP (TBMA), and finally with the self-management and learning elements integrated it became TBMA for self-management, leaning away from psychotherapy due to the greater understanding of the patients' mindset, avoiding mental health. Furthermore, it was clear a learning model would be far more suitable/

effective for this patient population which gives TBMA a uniqueness not found in other approaches.

After receiving ethical approval from the NHS and funding from the East of England Development Fund, Helen, together with a research assistant, promoted participant recruitment to the pilot study by presenting the study to various local general practitioners (GPs) surgeries. Health professionals did not really appreciate the term DMP unfortunately, and the patients referred were mostly those who had experienced dance as a child. One of the outcomes of the analysis of the pilot study interviews with patient participants in the study was how the intervention, then termed DMP, had supported a strong link between their body and their mind (Payne & Stott, 2010). Since the dance element in the term DMP was not favourably received by GPs for recruitment and patients made the connection between the movement of their body and their minds, a change in the label used to describe the approach emerged. This in turn led to a focus on learning as opposed to psychotherapy and key to this was self-management. Therefore, the intervention evolved organically developing its theory and practice in an action research model, each iteration informing the next. The title for the intervention of The BodyMind Approach therefore arose instead. Furthermore, it transpired people experiencing these symptoms mostly had a physical explanatory model, just not yet diagnosed. Many refused mental health interventions and were very wary of the term "therapy". Therefore, changing the title, underlying theoretical model and sessions to classes with embodied learning and an arts-based focus was more easily accepted by patients and health professionals. Furthermore, the classes did not aim for healing, mental health therapy or treatment per se, rather developing patient self-management. The term self-management is also more acceptable to the health professional community since patients are expected to take more responsibility for their care.

It is important to note the emphasis in TBMA is on the body first and foremost since the symptom/s patients experience are held in the body. However, the approach employs the symptom experience to reach the mind of the patient participant. Additionally, as there is no term for Body and Mind as an entity in the English language unlike in the German word "Liebe", the subjective body, the two words Body and Mind were joined together as one written as BodyMind, "Body" taking precedent and with a capital letter M in Mind. The term "BodyMind" for the classes was key since connections made between the participants' bodies and their minds were emphasised by them in the first pilot study (Payne & Stott, 2010). The term BodyMind Approach was crucial in distinguishing it from the emerging term "mind-body" which is now more commonly employed in health care.

We did not tell patients the intervention was called TBMA we simply emphasised the classes were learning more about their symptoms to make it more acceptable. In subsequent research studies the term "Symptoms Group" was employed as most patients and health referrers found this name for the intervention made it more understandable. This also led to greater accessibility. Subsequently, as adult learning became more embedded in the theoretical framework the classes were termed "Learning Groups" – learning more about your symptoms and how to manage them. These terms have proved to be more satisfactory to patients/GPs than employing nomenclature such as "mental health" or "therapy" (e.g., one patient recently stated at the beginning of a group "If this is to do with mental health then I am not staying!").

The second author originally suspected her MUS was happening as a response to stress in her environment but not a mental health condition. Much of the book stems from her keen interest in the physical manifestation of emotional distress. Her lived experience has been both as an insider and outsider to the topic. Her background is wide ranging Master's level knowledge covering the academic disciplines of human biology; education; social science and business. This provides her with a holistic overview of the theorising and delivery of TBMA. She has worked in a variety of settings including both secondary and higher education and the criminal justice system as both a practitioner and senior manager in a public service. Again, these experiences provide an overview of systems, group interaction and organisational dynamics. She was closely involved with the first author with the setting up, running and management of the spin out University of Hertfordshire company Pathways2Wellbeing. The research and dissemination of TBMA were additional aspects for which she was heavily involved.

Whilst TBMA intervention has its roots in embodied psychotherapy (namely dance movement psychotherapy) it is not a form of psychotherapy. It does not seek to explore or heal/integrate trauma, although it is trauma informed (for example, developmental trauma – see attachment chapter). Generally, the facilitators are trained psychotherapists experienced in group work but modify their approach to TBMA to focus on learning and self-management.

The intervention is designed to support patients with their MUS/BDD to self-manage their symptoms. The learning ecology (Siemens, 2007) in TBMA crosses borders between the arts, adult learning and health. This interfaces several major approaches that do not usually speak to one another. It takes place in a safe facilitated group with a focus on the symptom distress as a gateway to learning more about themselves and how to self-manage the symptom/s. It aims to overcome the obstacles of the patient mind-set about the symptoms, believing in a physical explanatory model, despite health professionals suggesting the symptoms are a result of mental health. Additionally, the lack of treatment options in both mental and physical health facilities leave the patient population with no hope for change.

The intervention was originally developed as a specialist, community-based programme (termed an MUS Clinic to GPs) for primary care patients with MUS based on research (Payne & Stott, 2010) and practice-based evidence (Payne, 2015, 2017a; Payne & Brooks, 2016, 2017), conducted at the University of Hertfordshire, United Kingdom. During the research a cost effectiveness study was conducted by a health economist to demonstrate the expected savings to primary care of implementing TBMA (Payne & Fordham, 2008). The subsequent delivery in the NHS was through a spin-out body (Pathways2Wellbeing) from the university, transferring knowledge for impact (Payne, 2017b).

Impact Statement

As a result of reading this book we anticipate health professionals who are working with people with MUS/BDD will have better guidance about how and when to use TBMA as an intervention in primary care available through either the National Health Service (NHS) in the UK, or abroad, or private health care. We hope policy makers, health professionals, writers and health bloggers will find this book useful.

The anticipated impact of implementing TBMA in health care could be:

- A change in how health professionals perceive people with MUS/BDD and their need for self-managed care (which can be found via TBMA groups).
- Health professionals in pain clinics, GP surgeries, A&E, hospital specialisms and mental health services will consider TBMA groups a pathway towards self-management for people experiencing MUS/BDD.
- Health professionals will need information about TBMA group deliveries, access to a trained facilitator, referral pathways set up and the argument for funding to be provided.
- Research previously undertaken demonstrates encouraging outcomes for patients with MUS. There is also an economic cost benefit model for estimated savings to primary and secondary care available which could be utilised.

Professionals who will be interested in the research include Integrated Care Boards (ICBs), GPs, wellbeing practitioners, arts psychotherapists, counsellors/psychotherapists, clinical psychologists, physiotherapists, specialist consultants, A&E, academics and GPs based in hospitals. They can all be involved in promoting the means for the delivery of TBMA groups through lobbying ICBs for funding. Barriers might include Cognitive Behaviour Therapy (CBT) practitioners as they might consider TBMA as a competitor to CBT services, although we acknowledge "many roads may lead to Rome".

Patients will be impacted as they will learn how to self-manage their chronic symptoms both bodily and emotionally. GPs in primary care will be impacted as these patients will not need to have so many appointments for their symptoms, freeing up precious time for GPs to see patients they can help.

Pain clinics, specialist consultants, wellbeing practitioners and clinical psychologists will receive fewer referrals for patients with MUS, freeing up time for them to offer appointments to those they can support effectively.

The ICBs will be impacted as the cost savings of investing in TBMA programmes can be reinvested into other health services.

Purpose of the Book

As well as informing health professionals, this book will provide suitably qualified practitioners with a step-by-step manualised protocol. The aim is to facilitate a group approach to self-management using TBMA with people experiencing chronic bodily symptoms, such symptoms may or may not have a medical diagnosis. Both groups experienced high levels of emotional distress interfering with day-to-day life. It will guide practitioners towards content for sessions, attitudes of mind, together with principles for practice to deliver this research-informed approach. The aim of TBMA is to address the whole person, holistically within a biopsychosocial model, each element of which will be explained in detail in the forthcoming chapters. The programme helps people to come to their own individual understanding of their condition, something which people with MUS often struggle to do.

What This Book Covers

The content of this book draws on previously published material, for example insecure attachment (Payne & Brooks, 2019), which has been updated. The book draws on both the qualitative and quantitative research studies (for example, Payne & Brooks, 2016; Payne & Brooks, 2020). Additionally, it builds on related works by other authors. For example, van der Kolk (2014) writing on mind, brain and body in the transformation of trauma and Maté (2003) on mental health in relation to psychosomatic conditions and the cost of hidden stress. However, there has also been a considerable amount of new theoretical material developed since the research was conducted by the authors.

The book discusses MUS/BDD definitions and terminology and its effects on patients. It considers the theory and principles of TBMA and gives the details of the programme for MUS patients. It explains the flexibility afforded to the facilitator by using content based on a themed approach designed to meet the needs of each group and guided by the facilitator's own professional training, expertise and skills in TBMA. The chapter on training facilitators covers the on-line programme content for each of the four training modules as well as the necessary mindset, attributes and competencies.

There may be repetition because some material in this book has previously been published, though it is updated here. Since each chapter can be read as standalone content some repetition is necessary and inevitable. Additionally, frequent changes in terminology mean that at times, throughout the book, these terms are explained. Nevertheless, we have endeavoured to make each chapter free-standing and understandable.

There are chapters on MUS/BDD; TBMA; The Programme; Training Facilitators; Qualitative Research; Attachment and MUS; TBMA, Student Stress and MUS; and Stress in MUS/BDD in Relation to TBMA. The epilogue brings everything together and offers suggestions for future research and practice.

The Audience

This book is essential reading for suitably qualified health professionals who are a TBMA facilitator or wish to train as one. They will require a background in adult groupwork and creative somatic practices and should be involved in supporting patients/clients in mental health services. Practitioners such as dance movement psychotherapists, and suitably qualified psychotherapists, counsellors, health coaches and counselling psychologists with an embodied background are all eligible for training. Practitioners working with patients/ clients experiencing chronic physical symptoms such as fatigue, fibromyalgia, IBS, backache, headache etc., for which there have been tests and scans returning negative for a medical, organic, diagnosis, will find the content enlightening and invaluable. Many health professionals will recognise patients/clients in this predicament and will also know that there are few interventions available. Many people with MUS and likely BDD do not engage with mental health services (CBT), because they do not believe that they have a mental health issue. Many are seeking a physical explanation for their bodily symptoms, which are both physically and emotionally distressing. Pain clinics and pharmaceutical medicines or physiotherapy do not support their emotional wellbeing and are often also rejected. Therefore, people with MUS keep returning to their GP or A&E for more investigations since the symptoms persist.

The programme fulfils both practitioners' needs for a protocol to work with these bodily symptoms as well as those of people experiencing such symptoms. Medically unexplained conditions are very debilitating and very common not only in Britain but world-wide. The lack of interventions which make sense to people with the condition and the fact that this leads to their disengagement from services, whilst continuing to pursue a quest for the cause of their symptoms, makes the condition very costly and difficult to treat. Equally, we theorise that the anxiety experienced by people diagnosed with BDD may also find support through TBMA, helping them to manage their stress response.

The book includes a detailed overview of the programme for delivering TBMA to groups. For trained facilitators and those wishing to train it gives a comprehensive summary of TBMA training course and the relevant research. For suitably qualified practitioners wishing to train in TBMA there are international on-line training courses which take place twice a year. As the training takes place online there are graduates from the courses all over the world who often ask for details of The BodyMind Approach programme and its delivery (which could be regarded as the manual for practice). The book is required reading and source material for trainees on the international TBMA training courses and for those who have completed the training.

For other health professionals it is illustrative of a programme which could be employed in their settings which offers acceptability and accessibility to patients with MUS/BDD. Since TBMA adopts an embodied perceptual learning approach based on biopsychosocial factors it can help many people without a medical diagnosis to make sense of their chronic condition at their own pace. This programme offers another way to engage people, who are generally hard-to-reach, experiencing unpleasant, debilitating and anxiety provoking symptoms.

How to Use This Book

As we have said, the book may be used by TBMA trainees to supplement their training experience. Additionally, it may inform other health professionals of the experiences of people suffering MUS/BDD and how an embodied approach to self-management seems to be acceptable to these hard-to-reach patients. It will inform GPs, physiotherapists, mental health professionals and others involved with the care of this patient population of the in-depth research undertaken, hopefully persuading them to employ a TBMA facilitator for their many patients. The book can be used as a resource for practices and sessions for TBMA-trained psychotherapists/counsellors working with individuals or groups of patients with MUS/BDD. Trained TBMA facilitators can use this book to refresh their understanding of TBMA for MUS/BDD self-management programmes. Each chapter stands on its own, so can be read separately from the other chapters. It is recommended the reader reads the introduction first then opens a chapter which most resonates with them.

How the Book Is Structured

The book is structured into ten chapters. A few are based on previously published material, completely updated and others are entirely new material. We now guide the reader towards each chapter with an overview of the contents.

This **Introduction** has provided the reader with a background to, and explanation of, the relationship between MUS and BDD and an introduction to the origins and development of TBMA. **Chapter 1** gives an insight to the adult learning theories on which TBMA is based. **Chapter 2**, entitled "An Overview of Medically Unexplained Symptoms/Body Distress Disorder", offers definitions of terms and an overview of relevant historical terminology. **Chapter 3** describes TBMA, its theory, principles, aims and underlying philosophy, as well as a comparison between CBT and TBMA, including a report on an economic analysis. **Chapter 4** provides an overview of TBMA as a group programme for delivery by practitioners. It includes programme administration, information provided to the referrer on the nature of TBMA groups, self-referral and GP/health professional referral forms and protocol. **Chapter 5** gives the reader insight into the training for TBMA facilitators. This covers the programme content and the ways in which the training is delivered in groups for each of the four modules of training, including mindset, attributes and requirements of facilitators. Several suggestions and examples of suitable forms for the implementation of TBMA groups are provided for facilitators.

Chapter 6 focuses on the qualitative research which rests on data from patient perceptions on their experience of TBMA programmes. **Chapter 7** illustrates how TBMA takes account of different types of insecure adult attachment and the link with MUS. It describes how TBMA is designed to ensure participants feel safe enough to engage with others and the content and to both bond with and remain in TBMA groups. **Chapter 8** explores how TBMA can be delivered in higher education to support students. **Chapter 9** presents the relationship between stress and MUS/BDD and how TBMA can interrupt this downward spiral. **Chapter 10** is the concluding chapter. Finally, there is a list of synonyms in the Appendix.

Next, we introduce adult learning theory as it forms the basis of The BodyMind Approach self-management model. Basing an intervention on learning theory is a unique approach in health services. The rationale for this approach is that some adults, and groups of adults, are more able to enter into learning situations than mental health treatment. It makes it more accessible as adults will have experienced learning in groups in education systems, however there may have been negative experiences from this. Learning in a facilitated supportive group with others with similar concerns, as opposed to individually, may give a sense of belonging and safety to enter and remain in the sessions.

Summary

This chapter has provided the reader with a background in medically unexplained symptoms/body distress disorder and TBMA, including its origins and development from both authors contributions. There followed an impact statement, the purpose of the book, what it covered, likely audience and how it could be used. An overview of the chapters showing how the material has been structured followed.

References

American Psychiatric Association, DSM5 Task Force. (2013). Diagnostic and Statistical Manual of Mental Disorders: DSM-5™ (5th edn.). American Psychiatric Publishing, Inc. https://doi.org/10.1176/appi.books.9780890425596

Creed, F., ... and White, P. (2010). Is there a better term than 'medically unexplained symptoms'? *Journal of Psychosomatic Research*, 68, 1, 5–8.

Edwards, T. M., ... and Kasney, L. M. (2010). Treatment of patients with MUS in primary care: review of literature. *Mental Health Fam. Med.*, 4, 209–221.

Pathways2Wellbeing. Qualified facilitators. https://www.herts.ac.uk/pathways2wellbeing/qualified-facilitators

Pathways2Wellbeing. https://www.herts.ac.uk/pathways2wellbeing

Payne, H., and Fordham, R. (2008). Group BodyMind Approach to medically unexplained symptoms: proof of concept and potential cost savings. Unpublished Report, East of England Development Authority and The University of Hertfordshire.

Payne, H. (2009a). Pilot study to evaluate Dance Movement Psychotherapy (the BodyMind Approach) in patients with medically unexplained symptoms: participant and facilitator perceptions and a summary discussion. *Body, Movement and Dance in Psychotherapy*, 4, 2, 77–94.

Payne, H. (2009b). Medically unexplained conditions and the BodyMind approach. *Counselling in Primary Care Review*, 10, 1, 6–8.

Payne, H. (2009c). The BodyMind Approach to psychotherapeutic groupwork with patients with medically unexplained symptoms: a review of the literature, description of approach and methodology selected for a pilot study. *European Journal for Counselling and Psychotherapy*, 11, 3, 287–310.

Payne, H., and Stott, D. (2010). Change in the moving BodyMind: Quantitative results from a pilot study on the use of the BodyMind approach (BMA) to psychotherapeutic group work with patients with medically unexplained symptoms (MUSs). *Counselling and Psychotherapy Research*, 10(4), 295–306. https://doi.org/10.1080/14733140903551645

Payne, H. (2015). The body speaks its mind: The BodyMind Approach® for patients with medically unexplained symptoms in primary care in England, *Arts in Psychotherapy*, 42, 19–27, https://doi.org/10.1016/j.aip.2014.12.011

Payne, H. (2017a). The BodyMind Approach™: Supporting the wellbeing of patients with chronic medically unexplained symptoms in primary health care in England. In: V. Karkou, S. Oliver and S. Lycouris (Eds). *The Oxford Handbook of Dance and Wellbeing*. Oxford University Press.

Payne, H. (2017b). Transferring research from a university to the United Kingdom National Health Service: the implications for impact. *Health Research Policy and Systems*, 15, 56. https://doi.org/10.1186/s12961-017-0219-3

Payne, H. (2025). Authentic Movement: A Culmination of Theory, Research and Practice. Routledge.

Payne, H., and Brooks, S. D. (2016). Clinical outcomes from the BodyMind Approach™ in the treatment of patients with medically unexplained symptoms in primary health care in England: practice-based evidence. *The Arts in Psychotherapy*, 47, 55–65.

Payne, H., and Brooks, S. (2017). Moving on: The BodyMind Approach for medically unexplained symptoms. *Public Mental Health*, 10, 1–9. doi: 10.1108/JPMH-10-2016-0052

Payne, H., and Brooks, S. D. (2019). Medically unexplained symptoms and attachment theory: The BodyMind Approach®. *Frontiers in Psychology*, *10*, 433131.

Payne, H., and Brooks, S. D. (2020). A qualitative study of the views of patients with medically unexplained symptoms on The BodyMind Approach®: employing embodied methods and arts practices for self-management. *Frontiers in Psychology*, 11, https://www.frontiersin.org/journals/psychology/articles/10.3389/fpsyg.2020.554566, doi:10.3389/fpsyg.2020.554566

Siemens, G. (2007). Connectivism: creating a learning ecology in distributed environments. In T. Hug (Ed.) *Didactics of Microlearning: Concepts, Discourses and Examples* (pp. 53–68). Munster Waxman.

van der Kolk, B. (2014). *The Body Keeps the Score*. Penguin Random House UK.

Chapter 1

Adult Learning Theory and The BodyMind Approach

Introduction

The BodyMind Approach (TBMA) model is based on adult learning theory and emphasises transformational, and experiential learning through its practices to support participant wellbeing and self-management of symptoms. For Bruner and Tajfel (1961), the purpose of education is to enable thinking and problem-solving skills, which can then be transferred to a range of situations. Adults bring with them a range of experiences and perceptions that can enhance or inhibit learning. Illeris (2007) argues that adults have resources that they can draw on in their learning and are motivated to engage in learning they see as having meaning.

Self-managed care/ways of coping with symptom distress may achieve specific goals. In the case of TBMA, adults engage voluntarily and will have the motivation to improve their quality of life in relation to their unexplained symptoms. However, negative past experiences of learning may bring barriers to engaging with TBMA that could be inhibitors to learning (Illeris, 2014; Wojecki, 2007). Some adults may see themselves as lacking agency in a learning context, so the learning process/context will need to build capacity and confidence in their identities as learners that they can learn, develop and change. Illeris (2007, p. 242) argues that when the hoped-for outcome of learning is a significant change and requires a readjustment or transformation in ideas or perceptions, then a person's learning identity can inhibit change ". . . even though the person wishes for it and is prepared to accept that the readjustments are necessary".

Learning in this context involves the development of skills, understanding and knowledge, as well as changes in perspective and identity that could be seen as transformative. This involves changing "our taken-for granted frames of reference" (Mezirow, 2000, p. 7) with the potential to think and act differently in the future. This type of learning is, as Illeris (2007, p. 47) points out, "extremely demanding and a strain and only takes place when the learner is in a situation with no other way out that can be experienced as sustainable". In the context of TBMA, participants are likely to be fairly desperate

DOI: 10.4324/9781003460749-2

for change and motivated to engage in this type of learning, although it may require a change in identity, from being defined by others and themselves in relation to the medicalisation of symptoms to someone who can develop a new story of their life whereby symptoms become normalised. Sarbin (2004) suggests that individuals develop their identities through story, and Bruner (1990) has focused on the importance of the self-narrative as a way of making meaning. An important aspect of what Ricoeur describes as "narrative identity" (cited in Wood, 2002) is that transforming one's story can lead to transforming oneself and "story revision" (McAdams, 1988, p. 18). The topics and practices employed in TBMA aim to enable participants to begin to change their stories in order to be more able to cope.

The methods used in TBMA have been designed to support participants through creating a psychologically safe space, which is vital if learners are to take the risks necessary to initiate change. Setting the group context is therefore very important. Learning is both individual and social, and group participants can both challenge and support. Challenge is necessary to engage in transformative learning as this requires critical reflection as part of the process. Brookfield (2017) stresses the importance of the role of others in helping to challenge assumptions and explore new possibilities. The group is also important as stories are embedded in cultures and fellow participants can help to challenge cultural stories related to well-being, wellness and illness. Agency (explored more fully in the section below on learning to self-manage), defined as the ability to influence events, is strongly influenced by self-efficacy beliefs that drive motivation and perseverance and influence achievement (Bandura, 1998). Agency can be bolstered by group members, provided the learning context is appropriately safe and facilitative.

Constructivist learning theory sees adults learning from the construction of the narrative of experience. People actively construct or make their own knowledge, and that reality is determined by their experiences as a learner. Whilst often undertaken through language, TBMA intervention also uses expressive movement/creative arts methods to access experience in ways that can help to safely challenge assumptions embedded in surrounding cultural discourses. This is likely to challenge participants in terms of their preconceived notions of learning and needs to be carefully structured in the class content and overall TBMA programme. The intervention also involves individual and group decision-making to facilitate agency and the taking control of learning. New skills, insights and perspectives should enable these adult learners to take more control of their own symptoms and to begin to re-story their lives.

Transformative Learning

Transformative learning, as defined by Mezirow (1997), refers to transformations of meaning (making meaning from the symptom during practices, perspectives, frames of reference and habits of mind, such as beliefs about symptoms) in which emotional and social conditions are important. In TBMA, there appears to be a transformation of perspectives, for example, from dependency, whereby the person's perception is from the symptom as the "enemy" to be removed by the health service, to one of self-responsibility, seeing the symptom as an "ally" whereby body compassion develops.

The importance of individual learning pathways (Mezirow, 1997) is acknowledged by TBMA. Each practice is undertaken with the participant "bearing their symptom in mind". Each journey will be different, yet a group closeness develops as participants witness each other's journeys. When considering transformative learning in TBMA, life experiences, feelings, beliefs, habits, mind-sets and lifestyle in relation to perceptions of the symptoms are appraised in the group, from which further learning can occur. For example, one person's goal at the outset was "I want to be able to clear out the understairs cupboard but my symptoms will not let me". The formulation that her symptoms prevented her achieving her goal had changed by the end of the workshops. She became aware that she had more mobility and more energy than she had previously experienced. She achieved her goal and cleared out that cupboard.

Dirkx, Mezirow and Cranton (2006) state transformative learning "suggests a more integrated and holistic understanding of our subjectivity, one that reflects the intellectual, emotional, [embodied, social,] moral, and spiritual dimensions of our being in the world" (p. 125). In TBMA, the subjective experience of the self and the bodily, sensory experience of symptoms are emphasised. Imaginative, social, emotive/embodied, intuitive, creative and expressive ways of being and knowing (McNiff, 1998, 2004) are therefore employed in a combination of education and consciousness-raising to promote self-management.

Transformation also points to a shift in the epistemological and ontological orientation of the person including a deeper awareness and recognition of the essential unity of mind and nature, self and other, in a participatory consciousness (Heshusius, 1994) representative of the transpersonal. Transformative learning through TBMA could lead to a more connected (i.e., linkages between sensory experience, perception, feeling and cognition) and more positive relationship between body, mind and other, providing a healthy platform for the self-management of symptoms. The unity of body (including the brain) and mind, which according to Siegel (2017) is both between and within us (in the person and between the person and the "other", whether nature, people, and so on), appears to be one outcome of TBMA. Comparing participants' and facilitator comments (from practice-based evidence such as evaluations and research interviews), Payne and Brooks (2019) indicate that the practices invite participants to reflect on subjective, personally experienced reality. Through unconscious and conscious processes, they make sense, create meaning, increase self-awareness and regulate emotions, within an open presence of mind.

Whilst learning theory can be critiqued for emphasising the cognitive rather than emotional, social and situated dimensions of the learning process (Illeris, 2004), the need for increased attention to the emotional dimension is well-established (see, e.g., Cranton, 2005; Dirkx, 2006; Kegan, 2000; Taylor & Cranton, 2009). Supported by this context, embodiment research has emerged as an interdisciplinary field, focusing on the complex interactions between bodily, cognitive and emotional processes (Niedenthal, 2007). Embodiment is the idea that knowledge is grounded in bodily states and in the brain's modality-specific systems (Niedenthal, 2007; Winkielman et al., 2015). From an embodied perspective, body posture and movement influences thinking, conclusions drawn and decisions reached.

Adult learners make sense or meaning out of their experiences (Mezirow, 2006). Social and emotional dimensions influence ways they construe that experience, and the dynamics involved in modifying meanings undergo changes when learners find them to be unhelpful (Mezirow, 1991). Tennant (2012) refers to the learning-self as the target for transformative learning. In TBMA, the consequence of this learning appears to be a new relationship with (or organization of) the self and perception and/or experience of bodily symptoms, which affects well-being, depression and anxiety.

Experiential Learning

Experiential learning theory defines learning as "the process whereby knowledge is created through the transformation of experience" (Kolb, 1984, p. 41). Learners build deep understanding and expertise through the four steps of the experiential learning cycle: concrete experience, reflective observation, abstract conceptualisation, and active experimentation (Kolb, Boyatzis & Mainemelis, 2002). Reflection in experiential learning includes personal experience, cognitive elements, feelings, emotions, meanings and interpretations from different perspectives (Fook & Gardner, 2007) – all these are present in TBMA.

Experiential learning is active and has its roots in the human potential for movement. Expressive movement is subjective in nature, fostering agency; where affect and emotion play a role in learning-by-doing, this is from the perspective of embodiment. Seaman et al. (2017) proposed revisiting the importance of the sociocultural context for learning (Sawyer, 2006) and the valuing of all experiences as embodied and situated as opposed to only utilised for abstract reflection aimed at self-understanding. Our body in movement is essentially how we experience the physical world – the basis for Kolb's (1984) experiential learning approach – where there is somatic interaction with the environment in which sensation, perception and cognition play a significant part.

Kolb's theory (1984) is not without criticism, for example, Rogers (1996) and Forrest (2004) contended the set of learning stages too simplistic and that several might occur at the same time. Jarvis (1987) and Tennant (1997) argued the theory was flawed because it does not account for global cultural differences, being largely a Western concept, and that claims made for the four learning styles were extravagant.

TBMA engages the learner in a process of knowing through the transformation of the concrete experience of moving creatively, reflecting on their own or witnessing others' movements, evaluating them, and forming new shared meanings (Vygotsky, 1986) about movement and the creative process. Subsequently, reengaging in active experimentation with those creative movements provides opportunities to assess their accurate communication and representation of the idea or feeling. These activities can challenge previously held assumptions (such as collaborative creativity) developing dispositions rather than absorbing facts or theories in the subject. Learning can become self-motivated, critically reflective and sustained independently (Perkins, 2008). "Action closes the learning cycle and reconnects the processing inside the brain with the world. It generates consequences there that create new connections that begin the cycle anew" (Zull, 2011, cited in Kolb, 2014, p. 142). Zull referred to changing the sensory experience into action; that is, from the sensory cortex to the adjoining cortex, and, through the reflecting/ thinking cortex, creating transformation.

Kolb (1984) tried to extend his model by the possibility for experiential learning to include somatic activities, but that unfinished effort resulted in several big philosophical questions, of which this review of some relevant literature seeks to illuminate by investigating how creative somatic activities may be understood as a form of experiential learning.

Kolb argued learning occurs when individuals (or groups) create knowledge through experiential transformation, which naturally involves the physical senses and movement, as we interact with others and environments. By embedding embodiment strategies, such as experiential learning (Kolb & Kolb, 2012), embodied practices can be valued without comparing bodies as in technical dance or competitive sports.

Experiential learning incorporates a "repertoire of learning instruments" involving body and mind (Claxton, 2015, p. 240). Thus, the corporeal experience informs and enables experiential learning. Experience here is perceived holistically, mediated by internal and external contexts, as theorised in grounded cognition theory (Barsalou, 2008). Recall is facilitated by partial/total replication of a learning situation due to relevant memory cues (visual, tactile, kinaesthetic). Sutherland (2013) suggested that in arts-based learning, meaning is made through emerging associations between the art object/activity and human interactions: an experience of "embodied selves in the moment" (p. 34) transitioning from "experiential learning to aesthetic knowing" (p. 25). Knowledge from expression through the body, viewed as experiential learning, can be constituted in phenomenological terms involving feeling, thought, imagination, sensation, sensitivity, corporal and relational experiences in a bidirectional process between body, brain and mind. The body "communicates social practices and cultural meanings through voice, gesture, and movement" (Cancienne & Snowber, 2003, p. 244) and dance, as a codified expression of the body, provides alternative embodied ways of making meaning/thinking and expressing knowledge.

Our body is not only functional – instrumental in getting us from a to b or an object to dress or get fit – but also subjective and expressive (Barr & Lewin, 1994; Bassetti, 2014). Our inner world of emotions, sensation, intuition, impulse, instinct, thought and imagination is reflected in how we move, gesture and take postures. We recognise and resonate, or not, with others through our bodies – their moods as reflected in their posture/movement. We consider it the process involved in the experiential learning of subjective experience, which is fundamental to both cognitive and emotional perspectives. The moving body as expressed through the subjective body (imaginative dance/movement play/improvisation) can realise and communicate thoughts, ideas (Bassetti, 2014) and feelings. When employing the concepts of experiential learning in TBMA there is immersion of the whole being in the activity, followed by reflection and evaluation of that activity, although not always necessary for learning through the body and sensation (embodied ways of knowing). Thereafter, active experimentation takes place.

This contrasts with the dominant discourse in Western education (Moore, 2004) which tends to view learning as mostly separate from physical and/or subjective experiences. When perceived as solely an intellectual activity, learning is in specific areas in the brain as a disembodied process, reflecting aspects of 17th-century Cartesian philosophy. Yet, experiencing the world is dependent on sensory perceptions of the body and the brain. Eisner (2002) argued concept formation begins with sensory experience and interactions among sensory modalities. Embodied learning arises from Merleau-Ponty's (Merleau-Ponty & Smith, 1962) phenomenological philosophy in which learners are viewed as within external and internal lived experience. The body mediates and shapes behaviour and ways of relating with others, artifacts and organisations (Kupers, 2008). This lived bodily knowing goes beyond tactile and kinaesthetic learning styles.

Preverbal expression continues once language has developed. Literacy involves translating movement expression and communication into words. The learning of language and movement expression is crucial to communication and understanding (Hanna, 2008; Kirsh, 2010). Peterson et al.'s (2015) integrated model for learning and moving links movement studies with experiential learning – it is thus supportive of the argument for experiences gained through TBMA to be framed as experiential learning. Here, the

Table 1.1 The Johari Window in Relation to MUS and TBMA

	Known to Self	*Not Known to Self*
Known to Others	**(1)** **Open Arena**	**(2)** **Blind Spot**
Not Known to Others	**(4)** **Façade**	**(3)** **Unknown**

concept of experiential learning is viewed as knowledge creation through the transformation of experience.

The Johari Window above is a communication model developed by American psychologists Joseph Luft and Harry Ingham (1955; 2001) and named "JOHARI" by combining their first names, Joseph and Harry. It is used as a tool for self-awareness training, personality development, interpersonal communication, team development, group dynamics and intergroup relations. It enables a way of looking at how we view ourselves as well as how others view us and can be used to open up communication with others. It may help to open up to others by sharing more information about us as we get to know them.

It highlights the ability to disclose or hide varying amounts of information about us. It also underlines the ability to receive or resist feedback about us from others. Hence it hints at the important issues of feeling safe and having constructive feedback to the concept of personal learning and behaviour change.

This model proposes four concepts: 1) known to self and known to others (open arena); 2) not known to self but known to others (blind spot); 3) not known to self, not known to others (unknown); and 4) not known to others but known to self (façade).

With reference to MUS, TBMA and adult learning this model can be viewed as follows:

1. Known to self and known to others: this refers to patient participants in TBMA groups and health professionals knowing the symptom experience. The patient knows their symptom experience and others in the group also know their own symptom experience, albeit differently. All is open to all. Patients are facilitated to move from the unknown to the known, i.e., the understanding of their symptom in relationship to themselves and self-management. TBMA group culture enables trust and safeness which both are essential for change. At the end of The BodyMind Approach programme it appears from the research that patients know more about their symptoms and how to manage them so known to self and others in the Johari Window.

2. Not known to self but known to others: TBMA group participants move through this model at different rates. Individuals may be in a position to learn from others' reflections on their symptoms and these others may have more insight than them so there can be learning generated from these group reflections. External motivation in TBMA can be seen when individuals might notice others moving from the blind spot into more a more open arena in that they feel seen by others and themselves. This can provoke another individual to leaning into more extrinsic motivation – e.g., "I see others preparing for change so I can change myself and gain the benefits I can see they have gained".

3. Not known to self or others: this could refer to the psychological understanding of the symptom sensation/experience and its meaning for them and their life management. Acceptance of the sensory experience has yet to be integrated into their understanding of the symptom. Both intrinsic and extrinsic motivations are present with this patient group. This relates to TBMA in that initially there is little external motivation although there is a lot of internal motivation to seek a cure and a diagnosis. This links to the Johari Window in that the patient is in the blind spot (they believe others will know and a diagnosis can be found but they do not know) (see top right of Table 5.1). Then following the outcomes of tests and scans being "normal" patients find an inner motivation to seek alternative treatments, supplements and self-medication such as vaping and/ or alcohol abuse. When the patient seeks help for their symptoms they are in the place of the unknown; they hope the health professional will be able to diagnose what is wrong but when they cannot the patient loses hope and faith in the professionals. The health professional also has the inner and extrinsic motivation to keep seeking a diagnosis so sends the patient for multiple tests and scans, yet all come back negative. It takes time for the professional to finally come to the understanding there is no organic cause. Their motivation is eroded and they say they do not know what is wrong. This is an uncomfortable place for both health professional and patient and fits the Johari Window of self and others not knowing.

4. Not known to others but known to self: this could refer to the specific symptom experience in the individual participant which is unknown to the experience of others in the group. It could also refer to the patient knowing the bodily experience of the symptom and the health professional not knowing. Patients may believe they have "the big C" but it just hasn't been discovered yet so they need more tests etc. This is the façade in the Johari Window, i.e., the individual knows but others do not. This can be interpreted as the inner motivation to keep seeking an answer. It is the belief that the patient knows what is wrong, but others are hopeless and cannot find the answer.

Each box in the window above could change size, expanding or reducing that area of knowing in accordance with the degree to which there "not knowing". It would be expected for example that the "blind spot" box might well shrink, enlarging the "open arena" box as participants move from "not knowing" to "knowing". Similarly, the "façade" box might shrink as the participants share reflections with each other and the group, thus expanding the "open arena" box again. The unknown box may reduce in size the more "knowing" develops either individually or as a group, again increasing the "open arena" box. Sensory experiences being a gateway to learning more about the self and life management result in the "unknown" window shrinking.

The Five Key Concepts of The BodyMind Approach Learning Model[1]

Participants are invited to be active in their learning. We extend an understanding of the success of TBMA as a tool for self-management through using the conceptual lenses offered by theories of adult, transformative and experiential learning. The five key concepts of such an approach are discussed below, namely: structure, agency, reflexivity, self-efficacy and self-regulation.

Learners are actively facilitated to learn to manage/control their symptoms. TBMA includes the learner's lived experience of their bodily symptoms, from which needs arise leading to goals being identified. The facilitated group environment provides a safe place for two vital elements for learning and new skill acquisition to take place. Firstly, there is ability to experiment with new ways of being in the body. Secondly, there is the important element of practising and gaining confidence to employ the bodily changes. Together these may lead to the dynamic of thinking differently about the body and the drive to practise even more, ultimately leading to a virtuous cycle of improvement.

Evaluation takes place at the end of the group workshops and, as the participant learner reflects in the group – with the facilitator and in her reflective learning journal – the capacity for self-direction is stimulated, supporting transformational learning (Mezirow, 1997). The pathway for each learner is individual. Life experiences, beliefs and lifestyle in relation to perceptions of symptoms are evaluated together from which transformational learning can occur. There is a focus on problem-solving in the context of the real, body-felt world of the patient participant. The objectives of the group depend on the themes and issues arising in the group at any one time as perceived by the facilitator.

Participants learn to take responsibility and develop confidence in their capacity to take appropriate action to resolve stressful situations in a changing environment. They learn to be openly communicative, creative and flexible as well as to incorporate more positive values. Participants may be given home practice, so they learn the strategies that can work for them, and are reproducible in different situations. This supports them once the group has ended and the six-month second phase helps them to stay on track with their action plan.

The five concepts of structure, agency, reflexivity, self-efficacy, and self-regulation allow us to conceptualise the processes underpinning the development of competent and sustained self-management of symptoms. Resilience in the face of life's adversities can thus be more effectively supported. We see these five concepts inherent in The BodyMind Approach model of transformative learning in symptom self-management as contributing fundamentally to the development of resilience. This is essential for managing symptoms post-group and independently, without the support of the facilitated group/health-care professionals.

1. Structure is generally used to describe societal arrangements, some of which are more fixed than others, which both arise from and influence individual action.
2. Agency refers to human beings' ability to act to change something.

The interplay between structure and agency therefore offers a useful explanatory framework for the efficacy of TBMA for learning self-management. Giddens's (1984) argument that structure and agency should be seen as complementary is supported by Bourdieu (1986). In this conception, humans draw on structures to act and, in acting, impact on these structures, often reproducing them. This understanding of agency allows for holistic consideration of our being in the world, which underpins transformative learning (Dirkx, Mezirow & Cranton, 2006). However, a deeper scrutiny of the context in which such learning takes place in the context of MUS/BDD suggests the need to problematise this view.[2] Here, the social structure of the medical profession wields a clear power over individuals, subjecting them to tests and labels, which may feel hard to challenge. Individuals are not wholly free to contest the systems (such as the NHS) in which they may find themselves and their agency is thus compromised. This compromising of agency remains an issue if, as Parker (2000) does, one constructs structure and agency as separate, with structures acting to constrain or enable individual actions. To support the transformation of habits of mind central to transformative learning and symptom control, the individual needs to overcome potentially constraining structures. In TBMA, individuals write/draw in a reflective journal during each session to help them to plan ways of addressing potentially constraining structures in the NHS. Enabling agency is key in individuals' lives and specifically in navigating health systems.

3. Reflexivity is different to reflection, which is thinking about, often in the past tense. Reflexivity is a more fluid, continuous, dynamic process of re-evaluation in the moment. Reflection and reflexivity respectively connect to Schon's (1983) concepts of reflection-on-action and reflection-in-action as tools to improve practice e.g. making a garden gate (trial and error, past and future focused). The feature of self-refection on action following TBMA practices to explore symptoms may lead to surfacing meanings and a greater understanding of the part participants themselves play in the existence of symptoms.

The ethnographer Tom Hertz (2007) claims that to be reflexive is to have an ongoing conversation about experience whilst at the same time living in the moment. Because TBMA emphasises the present moment, as in mindful movement for example, the participants will be encouraged to monitor their movement and sensory experience in the moment. This is a form of reflection-in-action (closer reflexivity, as a form of meta-cognition) which can lead to a lightbulb moment of realisation.

Reflexivity in TBMA refers to critical self-reflection on how the individual participant's background, assumptions, positioning and behaviour impact on their learning. This can lead to thoughtful, conscious self-awareness where participants engage in specific, self-aware analysis of their own role in their symptoms distress. This is not to judge or blame participants for their condition but to support their growing awareness of preparedness for change, the need for self/body compassion and acceptance of the situation (Payne & Brooks, 2020).

Reflexivity is a process of self-awareness through which we can critique our natural interpretation of life through reference to previous experience (Siraj-Blatchford & Siraj-Blatchford, 1997). Goffman (1959) conceptualises the reflexive process as drawing on a deeply held view of who we want to be, with actions judged by the degree to which they move us in the direction of this ideal self. In the case of people with MUS/BDD, this ideal self would clearly be one in which the impact of the symptoms was reduced. Archer's (2003) work adds to our understanding of the relationship between transformative learning and the efficacy of TBMA. Archer (2003) proposes that there is a reflexive process called "the internal conversation" (p. 9), which, she suggests, can act as a supporting mechanism for individuals in establishing a course of action. This internal conversation or inner dialogue allows an individual to increase control over their life/symptoms. In TBMA, reflexivity is enhanced through the verbalisation and journaling of, for example, thoughts, body sensations, feelings, insights, images and experiences during and at the end of each group workshop. A critique of this perspective might focus on the responsibility placed on individuals to chart their own course in a complex medical environment. However, it suggests that individuals can learn to self-manage difficult sets of symptoms. The concept of self-efficacy throws light on ways in which such a difficult endeavour might be managed.

4. Self-efficacy refers to an individual's belief in their ability to exert influence over outcomes, as with patient empowerment, which has been shown to be effective in the self-management of diabetes, asthma and other chronic conditions (Gibson et al., 2003). Self-efficacy affects an individual's functioning in four ways:
   - cognitively, through impacting on the degree to which people can plan for, and visualise success;
   - motivationally, with self-efficacy beliefs influencing effort expended to achieve goals;
   - affectively, with beliefs about potential success determining stress levels in attempting to achieve a goal; and
   - developmentally, in the avoidance of things we believe we cannot achieve and the subsequent inhibiting of life chances (Bandura, 1977).

Thus, what happens next is contingent on the degree of control we perceive ourselves to have over the future (Zimmerman, 2000).

Completing a task successfully could impact one's belief in one's ability to do it a second time. However, Pajares (1997) refutes this, citing research to demonstrate that the power of self-efficacy belief systems renders them a better determinant of future success than previous success. In the NHS there has been the experience of reducing patient's belief in self-managing their condition and being encouraged instead to accept this as a life-long condition which they have to "live with". In contrast, in TBMA, participants are encouraged to prepare for change and to believe it is possible to learn to self-manage their condition.

An association was demonstrated by Tsay and Healstead (2002) between patient empowerment, higher perceived self-efficacy and quality-of-life scores. Additionally, there is an association between highly perceived self-efficacy and increased communication, partnership, self-care and medication-adherence behaviours (Curtin et al., 2008). Empowerment of patients is an effective model of intervention used to facilitate quality of life, decision-making and self-care (Heidari et al., 2007).

In TBMA, participants are encouraged to be sensitive to the needs of their bodies, for comfort, movement and so on, and to give kind attention. The facilitator might ask if anyone would like a bolster for their feet in case the chair is too high. For example, after several sessions, a participant requested to sit away from a window due to a slight draught she felt on her skin. She explained she would never have cared enough to have stood up for her bodily needs like that in the past.

Through the process of TBMA, participants are encouraged to consider their learning from their symptoms to formulate an action plan to embrace following the group experience. This provides a sense of empowerment and the ability to take control of their future living with the symptom/s. Because the action plan is tailor-made from their own learning experiences they take ownership of it, giving a feeling of self-efficacy. The action plan is a living document, amended as required, and understanding grows or the life situation changes. This provides a sense of valuing their own experience and bodily wisdom, possibly boosting confidence and hope for the future.

5. Self-regulation involves the ways in which we control and manage ourselves, our emotions, inner resources, abilities and impulses. Self-regulation is the process of continuously monitoring progress toward a goal, checking outcomes, and redirecting unsuccessful efforts (Berk, 2003). An awareness of thought processes is required together with motivation to actively participate in learning processes (Zimmerman, 2001). It involves the learners' beliefs in their capability to engage in appropriate actions, thoughts, feelings and behaviours to pursue valuable goals, while self-monitoring and self-reflecting on their progress toward goal completion (Zimmerman, 2000).

Horne and Weinman (2002) proposed preliminary support for an extended self-regulatory model of treatment adherence that incorporated beliefs about treatment as well as illness perceptions. Self-regulation is essential to enabling resilience (Barlow, 2001) – the capacity to deal with adversity and to have the capability to recover quickly from change, stress or misfortune. Self-regulation is connected to self-management in which learning how to manage emotions to bring positive outcomes will either help or hinder progress. Through the various TBMA practices designed to enhance self-regulation, participants appear to learn to value their internal, subjective, lived bodily experience rather than seeing their body as an object to be fixed by another. Changes take place in both perception and action whereby a new habit is embodied, enabling them to take back control (thus developing resilience).

The concepts of structure, agency, reflexivity, self-efficacy and self-regulation provide a useful explanatory framework for the success of TBMA in supporting learners to be able to self-manage their MUS/BDD. These concepts can be seen to emerge from TBMA practices which support and cultivate extensions of them. The learner's experience both within themselves and between them and the environment, plus their goals in the individualised action plan enacted post-group are key. They draw on, and strengthen, individual agency. Self-management becomes embedded, as demonstrated in a six-month follow-up study (Payne & Brooks, 2016).

Learners begin to believe in their ability to effect a change in their situation and thus their motivation to do so is enhanced. They are helped to take responsibility for their own body and the symptoms affecting their day-to-day lives rather than depending on the medical profession. Home practice of specific exercises is encouraged so individuals learn the strategies that can work for them and are reproducible in different and unexpected situations. This supports them once the group has ended, and the six months of Phase 2 helps them to stay on track with their action plan.

Identifying a bodily sensation is the first step towards body awareness. Making sense of the sensation through various TBMA practices in terms of the relationship to it, the perception of its function etc., may lead to linking to emotion and expressing this in nonverbal formats. These practices provide signals as to emotional regulation needs and offer embodied changes to the bodily felt experience. Playing with the symptom engages participants in new insights into how the perception of the symptom can change depending on the practice. One prerequisite of successful emotion regulation is the awareness of emotional states, which in turn is associated with the awareness of bodily signals during interoceptive awareness (Füstös et al., 2013).

Tools for measuring emotional self-regulation do not appear to focus on the link between the brain-body and emotion. Emotions are based in, and expressed through, the body and movement. Accessing the body is a way in to accessing emotions (Michalak et al., 2009). Emotional regulation is fundamental to physical and psychological health, i.e., wellbeing (Aldao & Nolen-Hoeksema, 2012). In TBMA, practices which support emotional regulation include controlled breathing (Philippot et al., 2002); bodymindfulness and progressive relaxation (which reduces anxiety) (Manzoni et al., 2008) together with movement.

Consequently, emotional regulation is not merely a mental process but the result of an interplay between the body and mind. "Sensory-motor processes are not just side effects, but rather are vital in instantiating and regulating a desired emotional state, and thus to the effectiveness and efficiency of emotion regulation" (Veenstra et al., 2017, p. 1374).

For TBMA research studies to evaluate the outcomes of the intervention with reference to self-management, we selected proxy measures of emotional self-regulation using standardised tools. The measurement tools employed to assess changes in emotional self-regulation were PHQ9 for depression; GAD7 for generalised anxiety; GAF for general functioning; MYMOP2 for symptom distress and wellbeing; and data from these are collected and analysed at three time points – pre-course, post-course and at six-months follow up – according to reliable change criteria.

Summary

This chapter offered the reader an overview of adult learning theory on which TBMA is based, including transformational learning and experiential learning. Links were made between TBMA and MUS through examining the Johari Window conceptual framework. The five concepts of structure, agency, reflexivity, self-efficacy, and self-regulation allow us to conceptualise the processes underpinning the development of competent and sustained self-management of symptoms through TBMA.

Notes

1 This and the subsequent sections are based on the published article: Payne, Roberts & Jarvis (2019). The BodyMind Approach® as Transformative Learning to Promote Self-Management for Patients with Medically Unexplained Symptoms. *Transformative Education*, 18, 2. https://doi.org/10.1177/1541344619883892

2 Unfortunately, the abbreviation BDD is also used for body dysmorphic disorder which is a mental health condition where a person spends a lot of time worrying about perceived flaws in their appearance.

References

Aldao, A., and Nolen-Hoeksema, S. (2012). When are adaptive strategies most predictive of psychopathology? *Journal of Abnormal Psychology*, 121(1), 276.

Archer, M. S. (2003). *Structure, Agency, and the Internal Conversation*. Cambridge University Press.

Bandura, A. (1977). Self-efficacy: toward a unifying theory of behavioral change. *Psychological Review*, 84(2), 191.

Bandura, A. (1998). Personal and collective efficacy in human adaptation and change. *Advances in Psychological Science*, 1, 51–71.

Barlow, J. (2001). How to use education as an intervention in osteoarthritis. *Best Practice and Research Clinical Rheumatology*, 15(4), 545–558.

Barr, S., and Lewin, P. (1994). Learning movement: integrating kinaesthetic sense with cognitive skills. *Journal of Aesthetic Education*, 28(1), 83–94.

Barsalou, L. W. (2008). Grounded cognition. *Annu. Rev. Psychol.*, 59(1), 617–645.

Bassetti, C. (2014). The knowing body-in-action in performing arts: embodiment, experiential transformation, and intersubjectivity. In T. Zembylas (Ed). *Artistic Practices* (pp. 91–111). Routledge.

Berk, L. E. (2003). *Child Development*. Allyn and Bacon.

Bourdieu, P. (1986). *Distinction: A Social Critique of the Judgment of Taste*. Harvard University Press.

Brookfield, S. D. (2017). *Becoming a Critically Reflective Teacher*. John Wiley and Sons.

Bruner, J. (1990). Culture and human development: a new look. *Human Development*, 33(6), 344–355.

Bruner, J. S., and Tajfel, H. (1961). Cognitive risk and environmental change. *The Journal of Abnormal and Social Psychology*, 62(2), 231.

Cancienne, M. B., and Snowber, C. N. (2003). Writing rhythm: Movement as method. *Qualitative Inquiry*, 9(2), 237–253.

Claxton, G. (2015). *Intelligence in the Flesh: Why Your Mind Needs Your Body Much More Than It Thinks*. Yale University Press.

Cranton, P. (2005). A journey of heart and Mind: Transformative Jewish Learning in Adulthood. *Journal of Adult Theological Education*, 2(2), 182–183. https://doi.org/10.1179/ate.2.2.4501q61156l414r2

Curtin, R. B., ... and Klicko, K. (2008). Self-efficacy and self-management behaviours in patients with chronic kidney disease. *Advances in Kidney Disease and Health*, 15(2), 191–205.

Dirkx, J. M. (2006). Engaging Emotions in Adult Learning: A Jungian Perspective on Emotions and Transformative Learning. *New Directions for Adult and Continuing Education* 109, 15–26. DOI:10.1002/ace.204

Dirkx, J. M., Mezirow, J., and Cranton, P. (2006). Musings and Reflections on the Meaning, Context, and Process of Transformative Learning: A Dialogue Between John M. Dirkx and Jack Mezirow. *Journal of Transformative Education*, 4(2), 123–139. https://doi.org/10.1177/1541344606287503

Eisner, E. W. (2002). *The Arts and the Creation of Mind*. Yale University Press.

Fook, J., and Gardner, F. (2007). *Practising Critical Reflection: A Resource Handbook*. McGraw-Hill Education (UK).

Forrest, S. (2004). Learning and teaching: the reciprocal link. *The Journal of Continuing Education in Nursing*, 35(2), 74–79.

Füstös, J., ... and Pollatos, O. (2013) On the embodiment of emotion regulation: interoceptive awareness facilitates reappraisal, *Social Cognitive and Affective Neuroscience*, 8, 8, 911–917, https://doi.org/10.1093/scan/nss089

Gibson, G. P., Ram, F. S. F., Powell, H. (2003). Asthma Education. *Respiratory Medicine*, 97(9), 1036–1044. ISSN 0954-6111. https://doi.org/10.1016/S0954-6111(03)00134-3

Giddens, A. (1984). *The Constitution of Society: Outline of the Theory of Structuration*. University of California Press.

Goffman, E. (1959). The moral career of the mental patient. *Psychiatry*, 22(2), 123–142.

Hanna, J. L. (2008). A nonverbal language for imagining and learning: dance education in K–12 curriculum. *Educational Researcher*, 37(8), 491–506.

Heidari, M., ... and Moezzi, F. (2007). The effect of empowerment model on quality of life of diabetic adolescents. *Iranian Journal of Paediatrics*, 17(s1), 87–94.

Hertz, T. (2007). A group-specific measure of intergenerational persistence. Department of Economics, American University, Washington, DC, Working Paper 2007–16.

Heshusius, L. (1994). Freeing ourselves from objectivity: managing subjectivity or turning toward a participatory mode of consciousness? *Educational Researcher*, 23(3), 15–22.

Horne, R., and Weinman, J. (2002). Self-regulation and self-management in asthma: exploring the role of illness perceptions and treatment beliefs in explaining non-adherence to preventer medication. *Psychology and Health*, 17(1), 17–32.

Illeris, K. (2004). Transformative Learning in the Perspective of a Comprehensive Learning Theory. Journal of Transformative Education, 2(2), 79–89 https://doi.org/10.1177/1541344603262315

Illeris, K. (2007). What do we actually mean by experiential learning? *Human Resource Development Review*, 6(1), 84–95.

Illeris, K. (2014). Transformative learning and identity. *Journal of Transformative Education*, 12(2), 148–163.

Jarvis, P. (1987). Meaningful and meaningless experience: Towards an analysis of learning from life. *Adult Education Quarterly*, 37(3), 164–172.

Kegan R. (2000). What "form" transforms? A constructive-developmental perspective on transformational learning. In J. Mezirow and Associates (Eds.), *Learning as Transformation: Critical Perspectives on a Theory in Progress* (pp. 35–70). Jossey-Bass.

Kirsh, D. (2010). Thinking with the body. *Proceedings of the Annual Meeting of the Cognitive Science Society* (Vol. 32, No. 32).

Kolb, D. A. (2014). Experiential Learning Experience as the Source of Learning and Development. New Jersey FT Press.

Kolb, A. Y., and Kolb, D. A. (2012). Experiential learning theory. In N. M. Seel (Ed.), *Encyclopaedia of the Sciences of Learning*. Springer.

Kolb, D. A., Boyatzis, R. E., and Mainemelis, C. (2002). Experiential learning theory: Previous research and new directions. In R. J. Sternberg and L. F. Zhang (Eds.). *Perspectives on Cognitive, Learning, and Thinking Styles*. Lawrence Erlbaum.

Kolb, D. A. (1984). *Experiential Learning: Experience as the Source of Learning and Development*. Prentice Hall.

Kupers, W. (2008). Embodied "inter-learning" – an integral phenomenology of learning in and by organizations. *The Learning Organization*, 15(5), 388–408.

Luft, J. and Ingham, H. (1955). *The Johari Window: A Graphic Model for Interpersonal Relations*. University of California Western Training Lab.

Luft, J. and Ingham, H. (2001) *Johari Window concept*. http://postdoc.hms.harvard.edu/slides/AliceSapienzaJohariwindowmodel.pdf

Manzoni, G. M., Pagnini, F., Castelnuovo, G., and Molinari, E. (2008). Relaxation training for anxiety: a ten-years systematic review with meta-analysis. *BMC Psychiatry*, 8, 1–12.

McAdams, D. P. (1988). Biography, Narrative, and Lives: An Introduction. *Journal of Personality*, 56, 1, 1–18. https://doi.org/10.1111/j.1467-6494.1988.tb00460.x

McNiff, S. (1998). *Art-Based Research*. Jessica Kingsley Publishers.

McNiff, S. (2004). *Art Heals: How Creativity Cures the Soul*. Shambhala Publications.

Merleau-Ponty, M., and Smith, C. (1962). *Phenomenology of Perception* (Vol. 26). Routledge.

Mezirow, J. (1991). *Transformative Dimensions of Adult Learning*. Jossey-Bass.

Mezirow, J. (1997) Transformative Learning: Theory to Practice. *New Directions for Adult and Continuing Education*, 74, 5–12. http://dx.doi.org/10.1002/ace.7401

Mezirow, J. (2000). Learning to think like an adult. Core concepts of transformation theory. In J. Mezirow, and Associates (Eds.), *Learning as Transformation. Critical Perspectives on a Theory in Progress* (pp. 3–33). Jossey-Bass.

Mezirow, J. (2006). An overview on transformative learning. In P. Sutherland and J. Crowther (Eds), *Lifelong Learning: Concepts and Contexts* (pp. 90–105). Taylor and Francis.

Michalak, J., ... and Schulte, D. (2009). Embodiment of sadness and depression—gait patterns associated with dysphoric mood. *Psychosomatic Medicine*, 71(5), 580–587.

Moore, D. (2004). Curriculum at work: An educational perspective on the workplace as a learning environment. *Journal of Workplace Learning*, 16(6), 325–340.

Niedenthal, P. M. (2007) Embodying emotion. *Science*, 18, 316(5827), 1002–1005. doi: 10.1126/science.1136930

Pajares, F. (1997). Current directions in self-efficacy research. *Advances in Motivation and Achievement*, 10(149), 1–49.

Parker, J. (2000). *Structuration*. Open University Press.

Payne, H., and Brooks, S. D. M. (2016). Clinical outcomes from The BodyMind Approach™ in the treatment of patients with medically unexplained symptoms in primary health care in England: Practice-based evidence. *The Arts in Psychotherapy*, 47, 55–65. https://doi.org/10.1016/j.aip.2015.12.001

Payne, H., and Brooks, S. D. (2019). Medically unexplained symptoms and attachment theory: The BodyMind Approach®. *Frontiers in Psychology*, 10, Article 1818. https://doi.org/10.3389/fpsyg.2019.01818

Payne, H., and Brooks, S. (2020). A Qualitative Study of the Views of Patients With Medically Unexplained Symptoms on The BodyMind Approach®: Employing Embodied Methods and Arts Practices for Self-Management. Front. Psychol. Sec. Health Psychology, 11 - 2020 | https://doi.org/10.3389/fpsyg.2020.554566

Payne, H., Roberts, A., and Jarvis, J. (2019). The BodyMind Approach® as transformative learning to promote self-management for patients with medically unexplained symptoms. *Journal of Transformative Education*, 18(2), 114–137. https://doi.org/10.1177/1541344619883892

Perkins, D. (2008). Beyond understanding. In R. Land, J. H. F. Meyer and J. Smith (Eds), *Threshold Concepts within the Disciplines* (pp. 1–19). Brill.

Peterson, K., DeCato, L., and Kolb, D. A. (2015). Moving and Learning: Expanding Style and Increasing Flexibility. *Journal of Experiential Education*, 38(3), 228–244. doi: 10.1177/1053825914540836

Philippot, P., Chapelle, G., and Blairy, S. (2002). Respiratory feedback in the generation of emotion. *Cognition and Emotion*, 16(5), 605–627.

Rogers, A. (1996). *Teaching Adults* (2nd edn.). Open University Press.

Sarbin, T. R. (2004). A preface to the epistemology of identity. In C. Lightfoot, M. Chandler, and C. Lalonde (Eds), *Changing Conceptions of Psychological Life* (pp. 245–252). Psychology Press.

Sawyer, R. K. (2006). The new science of learning. *The Cambridge Handbook of the Learning Sciences*, 1, 18.

Schon, D. (1983) *The Reflective Practitioner*. Basic Books.

Seaman, J., Brown, M., and Quay, J. (2017). The evolution of experiential learning theory: Tracing lines of research in the JEE. *Journal of Experiential Education*, 40(4), NP1–NP21.

Siegel, D. J. (2017). *Mind: A Journey to the Heart of Being Human*. W. W. Norton.

Siraj-Blatchford, I., and Siraj-Blatchford, J. (1997). Reflexivity, Social Justice and Educational Research. *Cambridge Journal of Education*, 27(2), 235–248.

Sutherland, I. (2013). Arts-based methods in leadership development: Affording aesthetic workspaces, reflexivity and memories with momentum. *Management Learning*, 44(1), 25–43.

Taylor, E., and Cranton, P. (2009) (Eds) *A Handbook of Transformative Learning*. Jossey-Bass.

Tennant, M. (1997) *Psychology and Adult Learning (2nd edn)*. Routledge.

Tennant, M. (2012). *The Learning Self: Understanding the Potential of Transformation*. John Wiley and Sons. Inc.

Tsay, S. L., and Healstead, M. (2002). Self-care self-efficacy, depression, and quality of life among patients receiving haemodialysis in Taiwan. *International Journal of Nursing Studies*, 39(3), 245–251. https://doi.org/10.1016/s0020-7489(01)00030-x

Veenstra, L., Schneider, I. K., and Koole, S. L. (2017). Embodied mood regulation: the impact of body posture on mood recovery, negative thoughts, and mood-congruent recall. *Cognition and Emotion*, 31(7), 1361–1376.

Vygotsky, L. (1986). *Thought and Language (abridged from 1934b)*. MIT Press.

Winkielman, P., ... and Kavanagh, L. C. (2015). Embodiment of cognition and emotion. In M. Mikulincer, P. R. Shaver, E. Borgida, and J. A. Bargh (Eds), *APA Handbook of Personality and Social Psychology, Vol. 1. Attitudes and Social Cognition* (pp. 151–175). American Psychological Association.

Wojecki, A. (2007). Crafting youth work training: synergising theory and practice in an Australian VET environment. *Australian Journal of Adult Learning*, 47(2), 210–227.

Wood, D. (2002) (Ed.). *On Paul Ricœur* (pp. 15–33). Routledge.

Zimmerman, B. J. (2000). Self-Efficacy: An Essential Motive to Learn. *Contemporary Educational Psychology*, 25(1), 82–91. https://doi.org/10.1006/ceps.1999.1016

Zimmerman, B. J. (2001). Achieving academic excellence: a self-regulatory perspective. *The Pursuit of Excellence Through Education* (pp. 85–110). Routledge.

Zull, J. (2011). *From Brain to Mind Using Neuroscience to Guide Change in Education*. Stylus Publishing LL.

Chapter 2

Overview of Medically Unexplained Symptoms and Body Distress Disorder

Introduction

Immense pressure on costs is placed on both primary and secondary care services by medically unexplained symptoms (MUS) in the UK. It can account for 20–30% of primary care visits (Escobar, Hoyos-Nervi & Gara, 2002). These costs are due to the high number of GP/hospital visits and testing for an organic disease which is non-existent in MUS or treating a mis-diagnosed condition. For primary care, MUS has been estimated to be the fourth most costly population in the UK. Health service utilisation costs more than £3.1 billion, rising to £18 billion if absence from work, benefits and impact on quality of life is considered (Bermingham et al., 2010). Increasing life expectancy and rises in chronic illness, means MUS can become even more costly.

Day-to-day life experiences can be severely limited by these persistent, chronic physical symptoms causing excessive worry and discomfort. The search to find the biological causes for symptoms via many tests and scans is arduous and patients may feel they do not belong in organic medicine or alternatively they do belong, but a medical cause has not yet been found. They may feel disappointed and misunderstood by the medical model (Balabavonic & Hayton, 2020). Since MUS is an umbrella term for numerous conditions, charities, associations, support groups etc., serve individual labels only. There are no overall support systems for these conditions which are heterogeneous. This problem is a result of how the health service has approached MUS, dividing symptoms into many different systems of the body, for example, neurology, rheumatology, gastroenterology or none of these specialisms. People are sent to each of these specialisms for investigations, mostly tests and scans.

The National Institute for Health and Care Excellence (NICE) guidelines do not have recommendations for the treatment of MUS, however, there are guidelines for individual diagnoses, such as chronic pain (NICE, 2021), which includes psychological therapies with "Acceptance and Commitment Therapy" (Hayes et al., 2006) as the first-line recommendation followed by numerous other modalities for differing conditions found in MUS.

DOI: 10.4324/9781003460749-3

Although people with MUS are heterogenous, research shows shared characteristics, including a lower quality of life, reduced physical functioning and poor health, comorbid with mental health conditions such as anxiety and depression. However, the mental health co-morbid conditions are not the presenting issue for the patient. They have a physical sensation which is debilitating and for which they seek help. Furthermore, their explanatory model for their condition is physical rather than mental. Somatisation or psychosomatic are therefore unsuitable terms to describe this patient population. Very few accept a mental health referral or go once and then withdraw (Edwards et al., 2010). Many people experiencing MUS have a reluctance to embrace a psychological formulation, as proposed by Maunder and Hunter (2004) and Town et al. (2017).

Firstly, it is important to recognise there are many terms for the condition MUS. The term MUS is overarching (NHS, 2021) and used to capture several chronic conditions which currently do not appear to have an organic pathology (Kleinstäuber et al., 2015). Normally labels are given to these conditions such as fibromyalgia, chronic fatigue syndrome (CFS) / myalgic encephalomyelitis (ME), complex regional syndrome (CLP), irritable bowel syndrome (IBS) and others. This labelling may give patients some comfort. This patient group feel stigmatised (Nettleton et al., 2004) and are experienced by health professionals as challenging to treat.

Historically, these symptoms without an organic cause being found were originally called "hysteria" in women (Tasca et al., 2012). This derogatory term must have made women feel ashamed. Subsequently, the term psychosomatic conditions (Řiháček et al., 2022), still used in much of the world, stresses the psychological which comes first over the bodily experience which is regarded as secondary. This term implies that the bodily symptoms are unreal and imaginary and may have led health professionals to be sceptical about the physical symptoms and have led to pejorative, stigmatising labels such as "malingerers" and "frequent flyers" (Hatcher & Aroll, 2008).

There are many terms interchangeable with others including "somatic symptom disorder" (SSD) which is currently being used in the DSM5 as a psychiatric condition (American Psychiatric Association/APA, 2013). It is claimed the acronym SSD puts patients into one single group but acts as a reductionist label despite the heterogeneous symptoms (Mik-Meyer and Obling, 2012). However, the DSM5 says that the label attempts to stabilise expectations of sufferers. Perhaps this means the health professional's responses limits the patient's ability to change. In other words – "you just have to live with it". In the DSM5 the concept of somatoform disorder has been replaced by the concept SSD (APA, 2013).

Again, in psychiatry, the condition has been classified as "somatoform" or "functional disorder" (NHS, 2021). In the medical speciality of neurology, symptoms such as chronic headache with no medical explanation would then be called a "functional neurological condition" whereby overall functioning day-to-day is negatively affected by the headache. Alternatively, not being able to walk where examinations show there is no medical reason could also be called a functional neurological condition.

Medically unexplained physical symptoms (MUPS) are a more recent term which stresses the importance of the physical aspect of the condition. This change in terminology stresses the importance of the bodily element as opposed to the psychological. This may have had a positive effect on patients and health professionals in that it leads them away from the explanation being a psychological cause because no medical reason can be found. The psychological cause has been the default position.

Much more recently, the term "body distress disorder" (BDD) has been adopted as way of labelling these conditions in DSM5 (APA, 2013). It is defined as existing alongside an explained condition but emphasises the degree to which a patient's thoughts, feelings and behaviours about their somatic symptoms are disproportionate or excessive. Creed et al. (2010) criticises the term "medically unexplained symptoms" as limiting, burdensome and contributing to a dualistic view of mind and body resulting in a differentiation between organic and non-organic causation of disease. Those authors prefer the term body distress disorder. In our view a criticism could be that the word "distress" (emotional) and "disorder" (illness) makes it seem as though the condition is solely a psychological illness, requiring psychological treatment. However, despite this, we know patient's thoughts, feelings and behaviours around somatic symptoms, whether explained or not, can contribute to other distressing co-occurring bodily symptoms. It is counter-intuitive to be pro-active moving the body when in physical distress, although movement is often advocated by GPs these days. The physicality of the symptoms needs to be addressed as well as the overwhelming feelings about them. This is an additional benefit of TBMA since movement addresses the physicality as well as the emotional aspects of the symptoms, alleviating symptom distress.

The term "somatisation" found in the literature refers to the phenomenon of experiencing somatic or bodily distress in response to stress which is psychosocial (Lipowski, 1988). The philosopher Thomas Hanna (1988) defines somatics as the study of the human or bodily experience from within us. This refers to the subjective body and interoception (the feeling of internal signals in the body). The experiences found in MUS sit between the mental and physical health services. There is a clear bidirectionality between the body and the mind found in MUS. The phenomenologist, Merleau-Ponty (Merleau-Ponty & Smith, 1962) argues the body cannot be reduced simply to the level of disease without contemplating the importance of the mind and vice versa: the mind cannot exist without the body – the body shapes the mind (Gallagher, 2005). There are challenges to the proposed split between mind and body propounded by Cartesian philosophy (Willig, 2008) which formed the basis of modern Western medicine. The NHS continues to operate with a dualistic view of the mind and body (Dazzan & Barbui, 2015). Individual care pathways via specialisms (gastrointestinal, neurological) often lead to patients being treated as "parts", not as a whole person. People with MUS often have more than one symptom but because of the way the NHS is structured they are referred to many different specialisms with tests and scans returning negative results. This uses a lot of resources and may obscure the underlying cause of the condition.

Psychoanalysis, which is based on the medical model, views somatisation as a form of repressed internal conflict, or considers it to be an individual's struggle to symbolise their experience (Bronstein, 2011). Gestalt therapy from the humanistic school echoes this, suggesting somatisation results from the avoidance of emotional experiencing (Nemirinskiy, 2013). Interpersonal and mentalisation-based therapies align with these views and formulate somatisation as alexithymia and a deficit in mentalisation (Luyten et al. 2012). Alexithymia is when a person has difficulty experiencing, identifying and expressing emotions.

We know from research (Adshead & Guthrie, 2015) that some MUS patients have insecure attachment (see Chapter 7). There is a proposed psychological formulation for MUS based on a combination of attachment theory and existential psychology (Maunder & Hunter, 2004). This suggests an insecure attachment style (i.e. developmental trauma) with common features such as negative affect, increased anxiety and excessive help seeking. Insecure attachment can prevent the person feeling safe even when safety is available, due to down-regulated survival strategies. When coupled with unacknowledged death anxiety, it is believed to lead to obsession with the body and a hypervigilance of threat turned inwards towards the body (manifesting as somatic distress) for the purpose of monitoring internal signals (interoception) to avoid death.

Key to the cognitive behavioural therapy (CBT) model is how a patient thinks about bodily sensations, suggesting that benign sensations can be illness related and threatening to life, catastrophising, leading to panic attacks (Salkovskis et al., 2003). It employs predisposing, precipitating and perpetuating (Deary et al., 2007; Salkovskis et al., 2016; Sharpe et al., 1992) to alter negative cognitions or behaviours pre-determined by factors such as genetics or personality traits such as perfectionism believed to be maintained by a cycle of triggering and perpetuating factors such as stress or physical illness.

The term "medically unexplained symptoms" is therefore difficult to define. A suitable term which fits all parties, health professionals and patients is elusive, but the label MUS may drive the search for an explanation – hence unending tests and scans.

Notwithstanding criticisms of the term MUS, the medical profession reliably recognises this group of patients with bodily symptoms which appear to have no medical cause (Smith & Dwamena, 2007; Edwards et al., 2010).

People experiencing MUS share many characteristics, hence could be meaningfully classified together (Lacourt et al., 2013; McFarlane et al., 2008; Nimnuan et al., 2001). Although there has been criticism of the term MUS (Jadhakhan et al., 2022) it is acquiring traction again, and is still in use today, especially within psychological research and has been used for the purpose of this book.

The term "MUS" has received criticism as it suggests a classification based on exclusion and a newer term, "persistent physical symptoms", is preferred by patient groups (Marks & Hunter, 2015). In MUS a clinician decides whether symptoms have an organic cause or not based on clinical aetiology, examinations and investigations. Translating this into research settings has been problematic, and historically broad definitions have been required to encapsulate the scope of presentations in the clinical setting. Since Nettleton (2006), MUS has received more attention, and it has been routinely embedded in the literature.

The requirement for an exclusion of organic disease has been removed from DSM5 (APA, 2013) leading to the term BDD. In the "somatic symptom and related disorders" section, the focus is on the reaction to physical symptoms as opposed to the nature of the symptoms. Nevertheless, as most of the studies included in this book use the term MUS, we have retained its use for clarity whilst adding BDD which is representative of the ICD-11 diagnosis.

Research into Medically Unexplained Symptoms

The term MUS has been prevalent over many years and there are therefore plenty of studies employing this term. For example, in an early study, Kirmayer and Robbins (1991) instigated research into somatisation. They referred to unexplained physical symptoms manifesting in physiological systems and distinguished between "presenting" referring to anxiety, and depression referring to "functional".

In contrast the term BDD is new and has not been researched in the same way. The criteria for BDD may help towards making the diagnostic criteria clinically useful and it appears to be applicable across healthcare settings. However, there needs to be research studies employing the term BDD solely to provide outcomes which may be important to designing appropriate treatment programmes.

Pain experienced is subjective, as is the resulting distress, and will vary day-to-day. Many people experiencing MUS do have pain to various degrees, others will have different symptoms which, as yet, are unexplainable medically. Naturally, pain is likely to correspond with feelings of depression. Functional brain imaging studies have been conducted to determine the interaction between negative affect and cerebral pain processing. Fogel (2012) claims parts of the brain which activate in emotional or physical pain are the same.

A Cochrane review by van Dessel et al. (2014) reported on the effectiveness of non-pharmacological interventions to treat MUS and somatoform disorders. Results from the 21 studies indicated psychological therapies were superior to usual care or wait-list in reducing symptom severity, however the effect sizes were small. In comparing CBT and psychotherapy neither was found to be more effective. The evidence, though, was of low to moderate quality.

Differences in randomised controlled studies (RCT) of CBT with patients with MUS, with neither single nor double blinding of participants, permits the presence of confounding variables which could have introduced the Hawthorne effect or observer effects (Adair et al., 1989). In an RCT of CBT by Escobar et al. (2007) improvements in physical symptoms and depression were found in 60% of the population but waned over time. The RCT by Kleinstäuber et al. (2017) did find a significant decline in depression, anxiety, illness-anxiety and illness-behaviour but found no change in somatic symptom severity. Sitnikova et al. (2019) also showed an improvement in physical functioning and a decrease in pain over 12 months, but the effect sizes were not significant. Furthermore, measures for anxiety, depression and severity of symptoms across groups had no difference. Additionally, Sumathipala et al., (2008) demonstrated that CBT was no more or less effective than the standard structured care.

Kleinstäuber et al. (2011) conducted a meta-analysis using 27 studies of short-term psychotherapy for multiple MUS. The analysis revealed unsatisfactory effect sizes. For between-group studies, effect sizes were small but stable, and within-group analyses were mostly moderate. Koelen et al. (2014) conducted a meta-analysis of 16 studies, where the effect sizes for psychotherapy groups were large to moderate when compared to treatment as usual control conditions.

A meta-analysis by Menon et al. (2017) involving 11 trials in India and another by Liu et al. (2019) involving 15 trials in China assessed the efficacy of CBT for treating MUS. However, there was a low volume of high-quality research identified. Both analyses aimed to inform clinical practice and identify limitations within the current evidence. Both concluded that CBT was superior to usual-care, enhanced-care or waitlist conditions. They found CBT reduced somatic, anxiety and depressive symptoms, and made improvements in physical functioning. Effect sizes were small to moderate and social functioning was not significantly improved nor was the utilisation of healthcare reduced. Sumathipala (2007) included six systematic reviews examining the effect of psychological therapies on somatoform disorder. Results showed CBT was most efficacious in reducing physical distress, symptoms and disability compared with those receiving antidepressant treatment or other non-specific treatments.

An RCT by Kolk et al. (2004) examined the effect of a range of psychological therapies including CBT, client-centred and eclectic-therapy on MUS. Results demonstrated GP consultations and psychological symptoms significantly decreased during the length of the study, however, no difference was found in physical symptom reduction between arms. Differences between treatment modalities were not examined. The use of self-report questionnaires and the lack of blinding were also problems.

McRae et al. (2015) demonstrated with mixed-methods, that a CBT-only intervention may not be enough to help alleviate alexithymia and teach adult individuals in mental health services how to self-regulate their emotions. Qualitative semi-structured interviews of service users with MUS on 14 UK sites were conducted using thematic analysis. Insights into the barriers and facilitation of CBT were derived. The avoidance of psychiatric language prevented stigma towards mental health problems, which makes CBT more acceptable despite being in a mental health setting. These service users will already have made the links between their MUS and mental health, helping them to understand their symptoms as interactions between cognition and the body. Since the interviews were conducted with service deliverers, bias would probably have been present. There was also a conflict of interest as it was funded by the Department of Health. Geraghty and Scott (2020) offer a critique of CBT for MUS, suggesting the practitioners are only trained to work with MUS at a superficial level rather than at a deeper psychotherapeutic level.

Some research views MUS through a biopsychosocial lens, which aligns with DSM5 recommendations (APA, 2013). In this model the physical symptoms arise from interactions between biological, psychological and social factors (Payne & Brooks, 2017; Polakovská et al., 2023).

A mixed-methods study based on a biopsychosocial model conducted a non-randomised study of an intervention in the UK NHS (Payne, 2009; Payne & Stott, 2010). It used a 12-week group programme entitled "The BodyMind Approach" which integrated aspects from dance movement therapy (Meekums, 2002), authentic movement (Adler, 2002; Payne, 2025), mindfulness techniques and non-verbal forms of expression to explore bodily symptoms. A quantitative analysis on the self-report outcome measures was conducted as well as a separate analysis of qualitative interviews with participants compared with reports from the facilitator (Payne, 2009). The quantitative analysis demonstrated a significant reduction in symptom distress. The comparative analysis between participant and facilitator accounts, on the other hand, suggested congruence in the following areas: a) participants understood how life situations and emotions impacted their body as well as what may trigger symptoms; and b) the creative exploration enabled a greater connection between emotions (which were referred to as the "mind") and physical symptoms in the body as well as the impact of stress. In a later study (Payne & Brooks, 2016), participants went on to report enhanced symptom management strategies and a deeper understanding of the cause-effect relationship, where understanding the cause may mean some management over the effect. Criticisms of the study include a small sample size (N=

16) for the quantitative analysis as well as a lack of control group, allowing for the potential of placebo or Hawthorne effect.

There is research on training GPs to deliver psychoeducation to MUS patients (see Morton et al., 2015; Wortman et al., 2016). Outcomes were insignificant with small numbers. Patients were recruited via the GPs, introducing the potential for bias in the selection and the possibility of Hawthorne or placebo effect.

In conclusion, there are many quantitative studies for patients with MUS, however outcomes are inconclusive. There are a few qualitative studies, exploring other interventions such as mindfulness, which have been integrated into Chapter 6 of this book since the findings seem to overlap with those from TBMA research.

The quantitative paradigm which fits with the biomedical model is useful for making policy, manualising for further research and recommending treatment from evidence, but this evidence tends to be unhelpful for MUS/BDD patients who struggle with the mental health tag which accompanies CBT evidence. The embodiment of MUS manifests in the integration of body and mind, negating any split between them, and is a perfect example which requires a holistic response, in terms of theoretical understanding and treatment. Hence a biopsychosocial model is essential. Fundamental to TBMA is the valuing of the individual's subjective experience while emphasising the relevance of meaning and using phenomenological methods to understand the human experience. This chimes with the work of Corrie and Callahan (2000).

In a study by Rihácek and Čevelíček (2020) by the end of the programme there was relief which came from a perceived reduction in the impact of MUS rather than the modification of somatic symptoms. In support of this finding, many participants in TBMA studies reported their symptoms had lessened in impact on their functioning or completely disappeared.

Patients with MUS may be left feeling unseen and unheard, compounding feelings of isolation, frustration and possibly triggering deeper feelings of insecure attachment/not receiving attunement and care (Nettleton et al., 2004). Furthermore, GPs have their own prescriptive model with reference to referrals to secondary care in that they have knowledge of certain symptoms which could indicate a medical concern and thus make a recommendation to a specialism. If the specialism is not the answer, then the only possible explanation is that the symptoms are concerned with mental health. In the case of MUS these repeated consultations with no answer can lead to frustration for the GP in trying to meet the needs of patients (Howman et al., 2016). This failure of the GP to find an answer links to insecure attachment in MUS (see Chapter 7).

Summary

This chapter offered definitions of the terms medically unexplained symptoms and body distress disorder, the aetiology of these conditions and an overview of the research into MUS. The historical background of these terms was given – such as hysteria (in women), psychosomatic conditions, and functional disorders, alongside somatic symptom disorder. Later came medically unexplained symptoms in the DSM5, which is now termed body distress disorder. Each label for MUS says something about how the condition has been perceived by both practitioners and patients and the fact that it is found in many different medical specialities. The term BDD reflects the change from dualistic thinking (i.e., physical and mental health as separate) to a more integrated, holistic approach to the patient distress surrounding explained and unexplained symptoms.

References

Adair, J. G., Sharpe, D., and Huynh, C. (1989). Placebo, Hawthorne, and other artifact controls. *The Journal of Experimental Education*, 57(4), 341-355. https://doi:10.1080/00220973.1989.10806515

Adler, J. (2002). *Offering from the Conscious Body: The Discipline of Authentic Movement*. Inner Traditions Press.

Adshead, G., and Guthrie, E. (2015). The role of attachment in medically unexplained symptoms and long-term illness. *B. J. Psych Advances*, 21(3), 167–174. doi:10.1192/apt.bp.114.013045

American Psychiatric Association, DSM5 Task Force. (2013). *Diagnostic and Statistical Manual of Mental Disorders: DSM-5™* (5th edn.). American Psychiatric Publishing, Inc. https://doi.org/10.1176/appi.books.9780890425596

Balabanovic, J., and Hayton, P. (2020). Engaging patients with "medically unexplained symptoms" in psychological therapy: An integrative and transdiagnostic approach. *Psychology and Psychotherapy: Theory, Research and Practice*, 93(2), 347–366. https://doi.org/10.1111/papt.12213

Bermingham, S. L., Cohen, A., Hague, J., and Parsonage, M. (2010). The cost of somatisation among the working-age population in England for the year 2008–2009. *Mental Health in Family Medicine*, 7(2), 71.

Bronstein, C. (2011). On psychosomatics: The search for meaning. *The International Journal of Psychoanalysis*, 92(1), 173–195. https://doi.org/10.1111/j.1745-8315.2010.00388.x

Byrne, D. (2009) Complex realist and configurational approaches to cases. In D. Byrne and C. Ragin (Eds), *The Sage Handbook of Case-Based Methods* (pp. 101–113). Sage.

Corrie, S., and Callahan, M. M. (2000). A review of the scientist-practitioner model: reflections on its potential contribution to counselling psychology within the context of current health care trends. *Psychology and Psychotherapy*, 73, 413.

Creed, F., Guthrie, E., … and White, P. (2010). Is there a better term than "medically unexplained symptoms"? *Journal of Psychosomatic Research*, 68(1), 5–8. https://doi.org/10.1016/j.jpsychores.2009.09.004

Dazzan, P., and Barbui, C. (2015). From the 16th to the 21st century: how we approach mental health problems and where do we go next? *Epidemiology and Psychiatric Sciences*, 24(5), 365–367. https://doi.org/10.1017/S204579601500061X

Deary, I. J., Scott, S., and Wilson, J. A. (1997). Neuroticism, alexithymia and medically unexplained symptoms. *Personality and Individual Differences*, 22(4), 551–564. https://doi.org/10.1016/S0191-8869(96)00229-2

Edwards, T. M., Stern, A., ... and Kasney, L. M. (2010). The treatment of patients with medically unexplained symptoms in primary care: a review of the literature. *Mental Health in Family Medicine*, 7(4), 209–221.

Escobar, J. I., Hoyos-Nervi, C., and Gara, M. (2002). Medically unexplained physical symptoms in medical practice: a psychiatric perspective. *Environmental Health Perspectives*, 110(4), 631–636. https://doi.org/10.1289/ehp.02110s4631

Escobar, J. I., Gara, M. A., ... and Rodgers, D. (2007). Effectiveness of a time-limited cognitive behavior therapy type intervention among primary care patients with medically unexplained symptoms. *Annals of Family Medicine*, 5(4), 328–335. https://doi.org/10.1370/afm.702

Fogel, A. (2012). Emotional and physical pain activate similar brain regions. *Psychology Today*, 19(4).

Gallagher, S. (2005). *How the Body Shapes the Mind*. Clarendon Press. http://dx.doi.org/10.1093/0199271941.001.0001

Geraghty, K., and Scott, M. J. (2020). Treating medically unexplained symptoms via improving access to psychological therapy (IAPT): major limitations identified. *BMC Psychology*, 8(1), 1–11. https://doi.org/10.1186/s40359-020-0380-2

Hanna, T. L. (1988). *Somatics: Reawakening the Mind's Control of Movement, Flexibility, and Health*. Da Capo Press.

Hatcher, S., and Arroll, B. (2008). Assessment and management of medically unexplained symptoms. *BMJ*, 17, 336(7653), 1124–1128. doi: 10.1136/bmj.39554.592014.BE

Hayes, S. C., Luoma, J. B. ... and Lillis, J. (2006) Acceptance and commitment therapy: model, processes and outcomes. *Psychology Faculty Publications*, 101. https://scholarworks.gsu.edu/psych_facpub/101

Howman, M., Walters, K., ... and Buszewicz, M. (2016). "You kind of want to fix it don't you?" Exploring general practice trainees' experiences of managing patients with medically unexplained symptoms. *BMC Medical Education*, 16, 1–10. https://doi.org/10.1186/s12909-015-0523-y

Jadhakhan, F., Romeu, D., ... and Guthrie, E. (2022). Prevalence of medically unexplained symptoms in adults who are high users of healthcare services and magnitude of associated costs: a systematic review. *BMJ Open*, 12: e059971. doi:10.1136/bmjopen-2021-059971

Kirmayer, L. J., and Robbins, J. M. (1991). Three forms of somatisation in primary care: prevalence, co-occurrence, and sociodemographic characteristics. *Journal of Nervous and Mental Disease*, 179(11), 647–655. https://doi.org/10.1097/00005053-199111000-00001

Kleinstäuber, M., Gottschalk, J., ... and Rief, W. (2015). Enriching Cognitive Behavior Therapy with Emotion Regulation Training for Patients with Multiple Medically Unexplained Symptoms (ENCERT): Design and implementation of a multi-center, randomized, active-controlled trial. *Contemporary Clinical Trials*, 47, 54–63. https://doi.org/10.1016/j.cct.2015.12.003

Kleinstäuber, M., Lambert, M. J., and Hiller, W. (2017). Early response in cognitive-behavior therapy for syndromes of medically unexplained symptoms. *BMC Psychiatry*, 17(1), 195. https://doi.org/10.1186/s12888-017-1351-x

Kleinstäuber, M., Witthöft, M., and Hiller, W. (2011). Efficacy of short-term psychotherapy for multiple medically unexplained physical symptoms: A meta-analysis. *Clinical Psychology Review*, 31(1), 146–160. https://doi.org/10.1016/j.cpr.2010.09.001

Koelen, J., Houtveen, J. H., ... and Geenen, R. (2014). Effectiveness of psychotherapy for severe somatoform disorder: meta-analysis. *British Journal of Psychiatry*, 204(1), 12–19. https://doi.org/10.1192/bjp.bp.112.121830

Kolk, A. M. M., Schagen, S., and Hanewald, G. J. F. P. (2004). Multiple medically unexplained physical symptoms and health care utilization: Outcome of psychological intervention and patient-related predictors of change. *Journal of Psychosomatic Research*, 57(4), 379–389. https://doi.org/10.1016/j.jpsychores.2004.02.012

Lacourt, T., Houtveen, J., and van Doornen, L. (2013). Functional somatic syndromes, one or many?: an answer by cluster analysis. *Journal of Psychosomatic Research*, 74(1), 6–11. https://doi.org/10.1016/j.jpsychores.2012.09.013

Lipowski, Z. J. (1988). Somatization: the concept and its clinical application. *American Journal of Psychiatry*, 145(11), 1358–1368. https://doi.org/10.1176/ajp.145.11.1358

Liu, J., Gill, N. S., Teodorczuk, A., Li, Z., and Sun, J. (2019). The efficacy of cognitive behavioural therapy in somatoform disorders and medically unexplained physical symptoms: A meta-analysis of randomized controlled trials. *Journal of Affective Disorders*, 245, 98–112. https://doi.org/10.1016/j.jad.2018.10.114

Luyten, P., Van Houdenhove, B., ... and Fonagy, P. (2012). A mentalization-based approach to the understanding and treatment of functional somatic disorders. *Psychoanalytic Psychotherapy*, 26(2), 121–140. https://doi.org/10.1080/02668734.2012.678061

Marks, E. M., and Hunter, M. S. (2015). Medically unexplained symptoms: an acceptable term? *Br. J. Pain*, 9:10914. doi:10.1177/2049463714535372

Maunder, R., and Hunter, J. (2004). An integrated approach to the formulation and psychotherapy of medically unexplained symptoms: Meaning-and attachment-based intervention. *American Journal of Psychotherapy*, 58(1), 17–33. https://doi.org/10.1176/appi.psychotherapy.2004.58.1.17

McCrae., Correa, A ... & de Lusignan, S. (2015): Long-term conditions and medically unexplained symptoms: feasibility of cognitive behavioural interventions within the improving access to Psychological Therapies Programme, *Journal of Mental Health* http://dx.doi.org/10.3109/09638237.2015.1022254

McFarlane, A. C., Ellis, N., ... and Van Hooff, M. (2008). The conundrum of medically unexplained symptoms: questions to consider. *Psychosomatics*, 49(5), 369–377. https://doi.org/10.1176/appi.psy.49.5.369

Meekums, B. (2002). *Dance Movement Therapy: A Creative Psychotherapeutic Approach*. Sage.

Menon, V., Rajan, T. M., Kuppili, P. P., and Sarkar1, S. (2017). Cognitive Behavior Therapy for Medically Unexplained Symptoms: A Systematic Review and Meta-analysis of Published Controlled Trials. *Indian Journal of Psychological Medicine*, 39(4), 399–406. https://doi.org/10.4103/IJPSYM.IJPSYM_17_17

Merleau-Ponty, M., and Smith, C. (1962). *Phenomenology of Perception* (Vol. 26). Routledge.

Mik-Meyer, N., and Obling, A. R. (2012). The negotiation of the sick role: general practitioners' classification of patients with medically unexplained symptoms.

Sociology of Health and Illness, 34(7), 1025–1038. https://doi.org/10.1111/j.1467-9566.2011.01448.x

Morton, L., Elliott, A., ... and Burton, C. (2015). Developmental study of treatment fidelity, safety and acceptability of a Symptoms Clinic intervention delivered by General Practitioners to patients with multiple medically unexplained symptoms. *Journal of Psychosomatic Research*, 84, 37–43. https://10.1016/j.jpsychores.2016.03.008

Nettleton, S. (2006). "I just want permission to be ill": towards a sociology of medically unexplained symptoms. *Soc. Sci. Med.*; 62: 1167–78. doi:10.1016/j.socscimed.2005.07.030

Nettleton, S., O'Malley, L., Watt, I., and Duffey, P. (2004). Enigmatic illness: Narratives of patients who live with medically unexplained symptoms. *Social Theory and Health*, 2(1), 47–66. https://doi.org/10.1038/palgrave.sth.8700013

NICE. National Institute for Health and Care Excellence. (2021). Chronic pain (primary and secondary) in over 16s: assessment of all chronic pain and management of chronic primary pain. Retrieved from: www.nice.org.uk/guidance/ng193/resources/chronic-pain-primary-and-secondary-in-over-16s-assessment-of-all-chronic-pain-and-management-of-chronic-primary-pain-pdf-66142080468421

Nemirinskiy, O. (2013). Gestalt approach to psychosomatic disorders. Gestalt therapy in clinical practice: from psychopathology to the aesthetics of contact. In G. Francesetti, M. Gecele, and J. Roubal (Eds), *Gestalt Therapy in Clinical Practice* (pp. 573–587). Istituto de Gestalt.

NHS. National Health Service. (2021). *Medically Unexplained Symptoms*. www.nhs.uk/conditions/medically-unexplained-symptoms/

Nimnuan, C., Hotopf, M., and Wessely, S. (2001). Medically unexplained symptoms: an epidemiological study in seven specialities. *Journal of Psychosomatic Research*, 51(1), 361–367. https://doi.org/10.1016/S0022-3999(01)00223-9

Payne, H. (2009). Pilot study to evaluate Dance Movement Psychotherapy (the BodyMind Approach) in patients with medically unexplained symptoms: Participant and facilitator perceptions and a summary discussion. *Body, Movement and Dance in Psychotherapy*, 4(2), 77–94. https://doi.org/10.1080/17432970902918008

Payne, H. (2025). Authentic Movement: A Culmination of Theory, Research and Practice. Routledge

Payne, H. and Brooks, S. (2016). Clinical outcomes and cost benefits from The BodyMind Approach® for patients with medically unexplained symptoms in an English primary care setting: Practice-based evidence. *Arts in Psychotherapy*, 47, 55–65.

Payne, H., and Brooks, S. D. M. (2017). Moving on: the BodyMind Approach for medically unexplained symptoms. *Journal of Public Mental Health*, 16(2), 63–71. https://doi.org/10.1108/JPMH-10-2016-0052

Payne, H., and Stott, D. (2010). Change in the moving bodymind: quantitative results from a pilot study on the use of the BodyMind approach (BMA) to psychotherapeutic group work with patients with medically unexplained symptoms (MUS). *Counselling and Psychotherapy Research*, 10(4), 295–306. https://doi.org/10.1080/14733140903551645

Polakovská, L., Čevelíček, M., Roubal, J., and Riháček, T. (2023). Changes after multicomponent group-based treatment in patients with medically unexplained physical symptoms. *Counselling Psychology Quarterly*, 1-21. https://doi.org/10.1080/09515070.2022.2142200

Řiháček, T., and Čevelíček, M. (2020). Common therapeutic strategies in psychological treatments for medically unexplained somatic symptoms. *Psychotherapy Research*, 30(4), 532–545. https://doi.org/10.1080/10503307.2019.1645370

Rihaček, T., Čevelíček, M., ... and Roubal, J. (2022). Mechanisms of change in multicomponent group-based treatment for patients suffering from medically unexplained physical symptoms. *Psychotherapy Research*, 32(8), 1016–1033. https://doi.org/10.1080/10503307.2022.2061874

Salkovskis, P. M., Gregory, J. D., ... and Ólafsdóttir, S. (2016). Extending cognitive-behavioural theory and therapy to medically unexplained symptoms and long-term physical conditions: a hybrid transdiagnostic/problem specific approach. *Behaviour Change*, 33(4), 172–192. https://doi.org/10.1017/bec.2016.8

Salkovskis, P. M., Warwick, H. M., and Deale, A. C. (2003). Cognitive-Behavioral Treatment for Severe and Persistent Health Anxiety (Hypochondriasis). *Brief Treatment and Crisis Intervention*, 3(3). https://doi.org/10.1093/brief-treatment/mhg026

Sharpe, M., Hawton, K., Seagroatt, V., and Pasvol, G. (1992). Follow up of patients presenting with fatigue to an infectious diseases clinic. *British Medical Journal*, 305, 147–152.

Sitnikova, K., Leone, S. S., ... and van der Wouden, J. C. (2019). Effectiveness of a cognitive behavioural intervention for patients with undifferentiated somatoform disorder: Results from the CIPRUS cluster randomized controlled trial in primary care. *Journal of Psychosomatic Research*, 127, https://doi.org/10.1016/j.jpsychores.2019.109745

Smith, R. C., and Dwamena, F. C. (2007). Classification and diagnosis of patients with medically unexplained symptoms. *Journal of General Internal Medicine*, 22, 685–691. https://doi.org/10.1007/s11606-006-0067-2

Sumathipala, A. (2007). What is the evidence for the efficacy of treatments for somatoform disorders? A critical review of previous intervention studies. *Psychosomatic Medicine*, 69(9), 889–900. https://doi.org/10.1097/PSY.0b013e31815b5cf6

Sumathipala, A., Siribaddana, S., ... and Mann, A. H. (2008). Cognitive-behavioural therapy v. structured care for medically unexplained symptoms: randomised controlled trial. *The British Journal of Psychiatry*, 193(1), 51–59. https://doi.og/10.1192/bjp.bp.107.043190

Tasca, C., Rapetti, M., Carta, M. B., and Fadda, B. (2012). Women and hysteria in the history of mental health. *Clin. Pract. Epidemiol. Ment. Health*; 8: 110–9. doi: 10.2174/1745017901208010110.

Town, J. M., Lomax V., Abbass A. A., and Hardy G. (2017). The role of emotion in psychotherapeutic change for medically unexplained symptoms. *Psychother. Res.*, Epub Mar 13. 10.1080/10503307.2017.1300353

Van Dessel, N., den Boeft, M., ... and van Marwijk, H. W. J. (2014). Non-pharmacological interventions for somatoform disorders and medically unexplained physical symptoms (MUPS) in adults. *Cochrane Database of Systematic Reviews*, 11(11), CD011142. https://doi.org/10.1002/14651858.CD011142.pub2

Willig, C. (2008). *Introducing Qualitative Research in Psychology*, 2nd edn. McGraw-Hill.

Wortman, M. S. H., Lucassen, ... and Olde Hartman, T. C. (2016). Brief multimodal psychosomatic therapy in patients with medically unexplained symptoms: feasibility and treatment effects. *Family Practice*, 33(4), 346–353. https://doi.org/10.1093/fampra/cmw023

Chapter 3

The BodyMind Approach

Introduction

The BodyMind Approach (TBMA) has been developed from over several decades of study, research and practice specifically by Professor Helen Payne. It has been designed for people with chronic physical symptoms appearing in the body for which tests, scans etc., come back negative (have no medical explanation). These conditions were formally termed psychosomatic; but in this book we use the term medically unexplained symptoms (MUS) although we note these conditions are now within the umbrella diagnostic term body distress disorder (BDD) in the DSM5 (see Chapter 2 and see list of synonyms).

The biopsychosocial approach is fundamental to TBMA which integrates intervention strategies from the arts and different schools of body oriented psychological therapies such as breath-work, dance movement psychotherapy (authentic movement), mindfulness/sensory awareness practices and relaxation techniques. It uses group work as the method of delivery. Facilitated by a skilled, experienced and mindful practitioner, trained to a high standard in TBMA, it engages with the fundamental inter-relationship between body and mind, hence the title "The BodyMind Approach".

This approach is underpinned by the general principles of adult learning, mindfulness, the recovery model, attachment theory, neuroscience and humanistic psychology (with reference to the "skills for health" competencies). The overarching goal is to promote the self-management of symptoms for participants. The focus in TBMA is not only on symptom management through the embodied practices, attachment styles (see chapter 7), connection with the self and relationship with the body are also considered. Delivered in a community setting, TBMA provides for an interactive, group workshop model, informed by its pedagogical roots in adult learning and teaching, and with transformative, experiential self-directed learning at its heart (Payne, Roberts & Jarvis, 2020).

The terms employed for TBMA groups include "Learning Group" or "Symptoms Group" (learning more about your symptoms). These groups offer an experiential learning process for supporting participants with MUS/

DOI: 10.4324/9781003460749-4

BDD to self-manage their symptoms. It is not a technique. The approach honours the legitimacy of the participant's physical symptoms and identifies psychological and social factors needed for change to self-management. The body and mind notion is consistent with, and supported by, neurobiological models which draw on central nervous system mechanisms to explain MUS/BDD.

Multiple ways of knowing (Miller & Crabtree, 2005) incorporate a range of activities to engage patients in reflection and self-awareness, memories, body awareness, dance, body maps, improving body confidence and sensitivity, and enhancing self-care. Body stories of health and illness, and the complex relationship of bodies to life histories and context, are surfaced through the arts and expressive movement processes, rather than being solely verbal. As Swartz (2012, p. 21) says when referring to this form of health education, "patients challenge their own situated knowledge and transformation becomes possible". New and different practices, such as expressive movement together, result in assumptions about their body being questioned. Written reflections in participants' journals about their changing body experiences help develop insights and connected knowledge with their own and family/culture and collective knowledge. Through becoming more connected with their bodies, they can know the meanings of, and respond more appropriately to, bodily messages of pain etc. – for example, not rushing to the general practitioner or A&E but valuing, recognising and regulating emotions, thus benefiting them, and those around them. Furthermore, this helps people to be able to distinguish between the feeling of connection and disconnection with self and others.

There is a shared sense of agency in TBMA groups and participatory sense-making via the group process. Trevarthen and Hubley (1978) speak of the physical environment and social context as playing an important role in making understanding possible. Porges (2022) posits that it is embedded in humanity's DNA to seek feelings of safety, and the adequately safe environment's role in feelings of safety is crucial. Humanistic and experiential models (Panou & Baourda, 2024) are reflected in TBMA. For example, stressing the importance of the relationship with the facilitator built through the elements of validation, empathy and unconditional acceptance which help provide for a safe container. For feelings of safety, it is important to manage expectations from the outset whilst balancing this with hope for change.

Action-based (enactive) experiential learning methods are directed mainly towards affect-motor schemata which need not be understood cognitively. However, in TBMA participants are also encouraged to seek meaning from reflection on the practices which engage their sensory experiences. Johnson (2007) suggests meaning is grounded in bodily experiences. The process of making meaning operates through our embodied experiences, emotional encounters and sensory-motor responses. In TBMA, symptoms are explored and established modes of experiencing reconfigured, modifying ways of interacting with the self and the world. In relation to problematic patterns of regulation, participants learn and implement new more adaptive regulatory strategies. Cognitive, emotional, perceptual and physical aspects of self-experiences are inseparable and processed in parallel within the psychosocial context of the group.

The Biopsychosocial Model

The first point of contact for MUS/BDD sufferers is normally General Practitioners (GPs), who report feeling frustration with recurring consultations from patients with MUS (Howman et al. 2016). MUS patients, meanwhile, say consultations can leave them feeling uneasy with GPs who seem to misunderstand their needs (Houwen et al., 2017). Resistance to the biopsychosocial model emanates from a desire to categorise patients into either bio, psycho or social (Tavakoli, 2009). However, people, especially people with MUS/BDD, are complex, and a biopsychosocial model is more appropriate to represent this complexity.

Nevertheless, there are critical accounts of the biopsychosocial notion from a patient perspective (Turk & Gatchel, 2008; Geraghty & Esmail, 2016; Morone, Greco & Weiner, 2008; Shakespeare, 2006). A narrative review by Geraghty and Blease (2019) outlined the model's limitations in treating conditions such as chronic fatigue syndrome where patients felt it created opportunities for misdiagnosis and conflict. Frustrations experienced by patients wrongly categorised may result in less funding for example.

The biomedical model of illness (Farre & Rapley, 2017) does not consider the role of environmental, psychological or social influences accounting for illness; it bases itself upon solely biological factors and is the dominant model in Western medicine. Mental health services dismiss the body, and physical health treats the body in isolation. George Engel (1977) suggests a medical model offering a reductionist view of an individual's distress. He proposed a biopsychosocial model instead which considers the role of social, psychological and behavioural dimensions of illness. It is this biopsychosocial model which underpins TBMA.

The concept of mind-body dualism in the Cartesian paradigm assumes two distinct entities, the mind (which is not the brain), and the physical body (Damasio, 2006). Descartes believed the mind existed outside of the body, and the body could not think which led to the creation of two practices to the treatment of the mind and the body (Duncan, 2000). Health services are managed separately (mental and physical health), polarising the mind and body within health services and with patients (Caes, Orchard& Christie, 2017). By focusing solely on the bodily symptom, the increased body awareness has two possible outcomes. Being sensitive to it early on can then provide the signal to turn away (distract) from it or turn into the bodily experience. It is a choice, therefore. When turning into the bodily experience body awareness can be modified by mental processes such as attention, conditioning, attitudes, beliefs, interpretation, memories, appraisal and affect (Mehling et al., 2011). They take the phenomenological stance of body awareness as a combination of proprioception (awareness of movement and the position of the body) and interoception (sensing the internal state of the body) of which we are consciously aware. Body and mind are inextricably linked, enactive, embedded in the present.

The approach relies on somatic awareness, a normal part of consciousness, to resolve the body-mind dualism inherent in conventional multidisciplinary approaches. Somatic/bodily awareness has the potential to enhance understanding and conscious use of inner healing mechanisms at the basis of the placebo effect. This awareness also allows for a holistic application of the "biopsychosocial" model. The notion of starting with the "body/bio" is the neurophysiological manifestation of the symptom and a gateway to understanding biological, social and psychological factors held within the embodied experiences. "Psycho" refers to the (often co-morbid) psychological elements (i.e. anxiety and/or depression) and "social" encompasses the group and participants' family, work settings and society at large. It is the intersectionality between each of these elements which can reflect the complexity of the patient population.

The next section highlights elements of self-management in TBMA in the context of patients experiencing MUS/BDD.

The BodyMind Approach for Self-Management

Self-management here is defined as the ability to emotionally self-regulate and thus achieve living well with symptoms, especially at times of stress. The BodyMind Approach fosters the development of the knowledge, skills and confidence to become able to self-manage. This development is aided by peer support from other group members sharing their experiences. Relationships with the group and the facilitator build mutual acceptance and understanding in a safe environment. The group experience can help support other issues such as loneliness and low self-esteem. The group represents a resource of lived experience and shared issues for all members to draw upon and contribute to and which is accessible and inclusive. Relaxation and general management strategies play a large role in self-management as demonstrated in a systematic review by Pourová et al. (2020) both of which are incorporated in TBMA.

Research has demonstrated there are more successful outcomes for people with MUS when strategies have encouraged the development of body awareness and the regulation of autonomic arousal (Calsius et al., 2016). Observing the physical effects of emotional experiencing and its connection to somatic symptoms is key to connecting body with mind or, as described by others, 'mind-body connections' (Pourová et al., 2020; Řiháček & Čevelíček 2020; Town et al., 2019). These connections between emotional states and somatic experiences are inconsistent for MUS sufferers (Town et al., 2019), hence the need for a biopsychosocial (see above) formulation.

Self-management requires the courage to take responsibility for changing the status quo and doing things differently. It gives the freedom to make choices about what to do and what not to do. It develops a feeling of accountability to self for actions. It gives permission to have agency and control over one's own life. Whilst this may sound an obvious statement, for people with MUS/BDD it is a life changing, lightbulb moment. This is because they have often come to regard themselves as disabled and restricted by their condition. Additionally, they may have experienced the isolation of feeling that they are the only one who has a symptom for which no medical diagnosis can be found. It becomes empowering to be able to take part in their own action planning for the future.

In TBMA each participant charts their own path to recovery through their action plan. Participants in TBMA appear to experience freedom of emotional expression through a variety of arts-based and movement practices. This can lead to an internal adjustment resulting in empowerment and the self-management of symptoms. Participants are their own expert by experience and their action plan is based on their understanding of themselves via their symptom sensations in the practices. This attitude of mind cultivates feelings of empowerment, novel for this population, enabling them to reduce health service visits.

Despite MUS/BDD sufferers being experienced as challenging and expensive to treat, these obstacles can be overcome with TBMA. That is, TBMA engages patients and is less costly than constant tests and scans, GP visits etc. The BodyMind Approach research demonstrates participants once engaged are willing to begin recovery through their capacity to identify a recovery and symptom management pathway central to their unique needs.

An aging population, longer life spans and more people living with long term conditions are becoming a burden on an already over-stretched health service. Therefore, patients are expected to take more responsibility for their own care in the NHS according to the United Kingdom Expert Patient Programme. Patients need to learn to manage the complex psychosocial issues arising from their condition. Self-management may be crucial to closing the gap between patient needs and health service capacity (Barlow et al., 2002). Emotional self-regulation (Barlow, 2001) is crucial to resilience; life will continue to generate stresses for patients who may experience their symptoms even more as a result if they cannot manage stress effectively. Learning about the possible stress responses as they occur in the BodyMind can be helpful to understand their bodily reactions.

There do not appear to have been interventions aimed at improving self-management for this long-term condition, unlike for asthma or diabetes for example, according to a Cochrane Review (Gibson et al., 2003). Purdy (2010) found self-management reduced unplanned hospital admissions for chronic obstructive pulmonary disease and asthma. Bjørnnes et al. (2018) in a meta-summary of qualitative research of self-management for women with cardiac pain found support for an individualised intervention strategy. This promoted goal setting, action planning, managing physical and emotional responses, and social facilitation. The model in TBMA satisfies these findings through a facilitated group self-management programme with individual goal setting and action plans for people with MUS/BDD. It emphasises multiple ways of knowing, social facilitation and managing physical and emotional responses. Addressing the long-term aim of self-managing symptoms in a sustainable manner reduces the gap between patient needs and funding constraints. A Cochrane Collaboration Review examined the more rigorously tested interventions to improve primary care for diabetes, another long-term chronic condition, and included the conclusion that patient-oriented interventions of an educational or supportive nature were amongst successful approaches (Renders et al., 2001). This confirms earlier literature that states chronic disease interventions positively affecting patient wellbeing necessarily include systematic efforts to increase patients' knowledge, skills and confidence to manage their condition (Von Korff et al., 1997). Traditional patient education emphasised knowledge acquisition and didactic classroom teaching. While such interventions increased knowledge, they were unsuccessful in changing behaviour or improving disease control and other outcomes (Clement et al., 2005). Nevertheless, confidence in manging the condition improved when adding skills to their knowledge (Norris et al., 2001). The BodyMind Approach model reinforces the patient's crucial role in managing the condition, helping them to experience their body in different ways and circumstances, and to be curious about the symptom/s. From the experimentation during the practices, they may develop goals for improving their self-management, identifying any barriers to them by designing a self-management action plan to carry out actions to reach those goals. Woolf et al. (1999) recommend supportive reminder systems to reinforce the plan which TBMA programmes undertake.

Educational interventions have been commonly used as strategies to improve health outcomes of patients with low health literacy (Schaefer, 2008). Studies have found health education may improve patients' knowledge and treatment of a disease leading to better treatment adherence and patients taking a more positive role in the management of their health (Shaw & Bosworth, 2012). Additionally, changes to lifestyle and increased adherence to antihypertensive medications to improve effective blood pressure control in hypertensive patients have been found (Meyer et al., 1985). Research concluded that interactive education workshops may be the most effective strategy in community-based health promotion education programmes for hypertensive patients; they improved patients' knowledge on hypertension and alleviated clinical risk factors, preventing hypertension-related complications (Lu et al., 2015). Consequently, it can be argued that an interactive, workshop learning model may be helpful in supporting patients with MUS/BDD to self-manage their condition.

Many MUS/BDD patients have different mind-sets so require different interventions (Payne & Brooks, 2018). As a different intervention, TBMA engages patients by working directly with their symptoms rather than from the mental faculty. In addressing this resistance to engagement in mental health, TBMA is framed as a learning approach not a treatment or psychological therapy for mental health. However, once engaged in a process this can promote feelings of control and self-management for participants.

The aim of TBMA is to promote self-management so participants can live well with their symptoms day-to-day – so, as one participant explained, "the bad days are not so bad anymore". Participants come with a lack of confidence, downtrodden and feeling inept. They feel disempowered due to the time spent in the health system searching for an explanation which cannot be found.

In TBMA, self-responsibility is encouraged, and self-directedness is inherent in setting realistic, relevant goals and helping participants to learn how to manage symptoms emphasising the learner's lived experience of their bodily symptoms. The most consistent positive outcome of interventions to improve self-care has been improvement in self-efficacy (Bandura, 1977), an important element of self-management.

Figure 3.1 below shows the intersectionality between transformative and adult learning theories which feed into the processes inherent in TBMA, which form the basis for developing the resilience required for competent self-management (Payne, Roberts & Jarvis, 2020).

Self-management involves the principles of adult learning, whether combined or not with biological, psychological and social interventions, treatments or techniques. The overall aim is to maximise the emotional self-regulatory function of the individual patient. Empowering people to be confident in their ability and capacity to care for themselves reduces the impact of the condition on day-to-day functioning and prevents the impact increasing.

Self-management in healthcare is defined in different ways, incorporating prevention and decline. It aims to increase the capacity for self-regulation monitoring thoughts, sensations, feelings and behaviours. The impact of self-management groups has the potential to improve health outcomes, such as increases in patient confidence and physical functioning, adherence to treatment/medication and reduction of anxiety (Challis et al., 2010).

Theoretical Overview

Figure 3.2 below illustrates the model and the key elements which comprise it and which are discussed at various places in this chapter.

Several key areas of research have been integral to the development of The BodyMind Approach model. Figure 3.3 below shows the research upon which TBMA has drawn. Each area is discussed in the book, such as in the

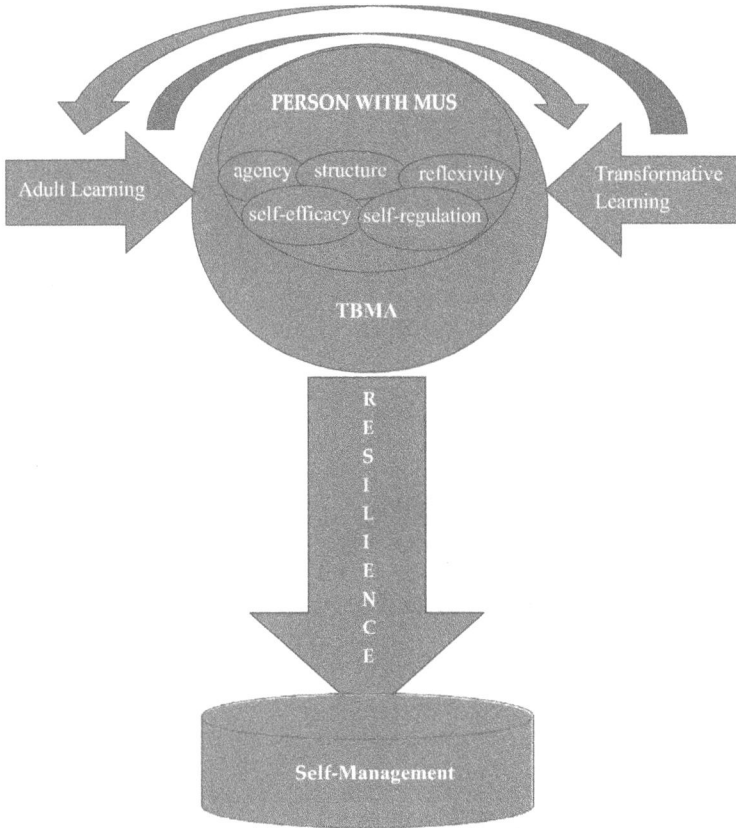

Figure 3.1 Showing the links between transformative and adult learning theories which feed into the processes inherent in TBMA

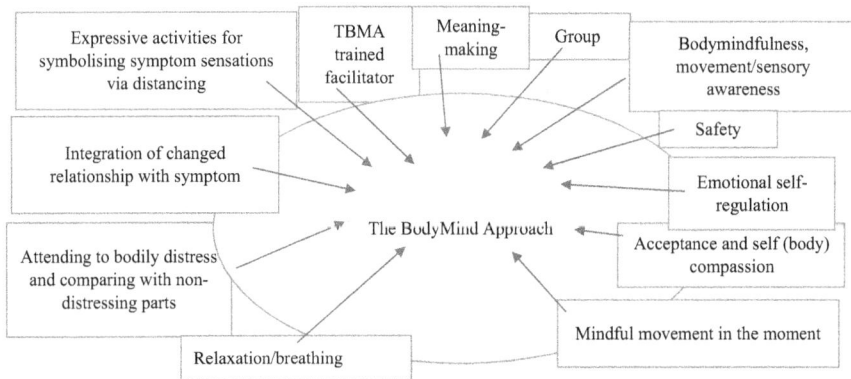

Figure 3.2 Showing The BodyMind Approach Model

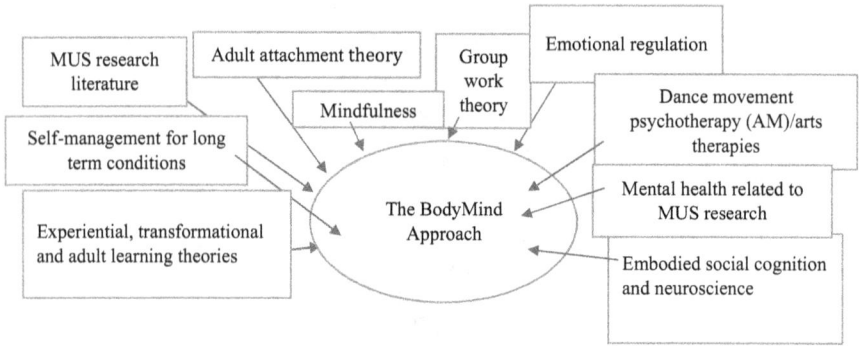

Figure 3.3   The conceptual framework for TBMA

introduction, in the overview of medically unexplained symptoms chapter, in the attachment theory chapter or in this chapter.

Changes occur via TBMA in, for example, symptom perception; relationship with the symptom; feelings of isolation; wellbeing; coping styles; illness and wellness beliefs; medication/GP dependence; and personal dynamics necessary to achieve a reduction in symptom distress and an increase in the feeling of control. The learning derived from TBMA extends beyond the acquisition of information for participants. It involves a deep understanding of the connection between body, thoughts, emotions, behaviours and the interconnectedness of these elements within the environment. Through this process participants acquire valuable insights into causes of their bodily challenges, develop management strategies, and enhance emotional regulation. They learn tailor-made practical skills for managing their symptoms, stress, communication and the fostering of healthier relationships. As a form of experiential learning individuals actively engage with, and reflect on both internal (through feelings, imagination, sensory and interoception awareness) and external worlds.

The reason we term TBMA a "learning" or "symptoms" group to participants and referrers is due to the stigma associated with the terms "mental health", "psychotherapy", "counselling" or "psychological therapies". This stigma is significantly reduced, enabling many more people from this hard-to-reach group access to this supportive intervention, most of whom would not otherwise entertain the idea of any link between body and mind.

Many participants have had their symptoms for several years and the chronicity has left them with little hope for change. They do not want to accept or access psychological therapies as they believe and experience the symptom solely in their body. They do not wish to go through the mental health door as they do not see themselves having a mental health problem.

The focus in TBMA groups, at least initially, is on wellbeing issues and more of an emphasis on understanding their symptoms from the outside in rather than the inside out. This enables the participant to firstly, access the classes and, secondly, by addressing the sensory/physical symptom this enables the participant to dwell within the symptom with a degree of acceptance, learning to live well with the symptom. Eventually there emerges a new understanding from the inside out of fresh coping, self-management strategies whereby the participant feels more in control. The symptom becomes an ally rather than an enemy since the sensation of the symptom flags the need for self-management.

Underlying Philosophical Values of The BodyMind Approach

First and foremost, TBMA takes an integrated holistic view of "BodyMind" interactions and moves away from the dualistic thinking employed in the separation of mind and body reflected in mental health and physical health services. Hence the body is seen as a gateway to understanding and accessing mind-body interactions and a deeper knowledge of the self. This gateway is free from the stigma and shame associated with mental health and is therefore often more readily acceptable to patients. As part of this holistic view TBMA uses a biopsychosocial approach, integrating knowledge of physical, psychological and social aspects of life.

The BodyMind Approach adopts the social model of disability developed by disabled people rather than the medical model. It describes people as being disabled by barriers in society rather than by impairment or difference. Barriers can involve the physical environment, people's attitudes, the way people communicate, how institutions and organisations are run and how society discriminates against people who are perceived as different, hence if society was structed in a way that was accessible for disabled people they would not be excluded or restricted. In TBMA equality, equity and inclusion are adopted which is important for the MUS/BDD population since they often experience isolation. The group experience provides a safe environment to support individuals and can also promote independence, choice and control. The model utilises the patient's strengths and resources rather than focusing on remediation and deficits.

There is no recipe or rigid programme-prescribed pathway for delivery of TBMA. It rather relies on the flexibility, creativity and professional training of skilled facilitators to judge the needs for a group/individual rather than forcing a "one size fits all" approach on participants who may have different needs. The manual provides content based on a themed approach designed to meet the needs of each individual group, guided by the facilitator's own previous professional expertise and skills. Facilitators are previously trained to Master's level in a relevant health profession therefore do not need an instruction manual but guidance and protocols. The mind-set of facilitators is nurtured for this population and the facilitation style of practice empowers self-managed care. For example, in TBMA the symptom is validated as opposed to other approaches which invalidate and negate the symptom. Terms such as psychological therapies/psychosomatic conditions can stigmatise and alienate people experiencing MUS/BDD.

Groups take place in a non-medical venue in the community designed to be more anonymous than a GP surgery/psychological services to avoid the shame and stigma that people may feel associated with attending mental health services. The groups are described as Symptoms or Learning Groups to patients and consider lifestyle, goals and action planning. This practical approach to the symptom focuses the attention of participants on issues that they can change to help themselves and gains traction with practice. A variety of creative, expressive methods are used including embodied experiences which focus on the sensory experience of the symptom and afford the opportunity for participants to develop a new understanding of the symptom and its meaning in their lives.

The process starts where the patient is: accepting the importance of the physical, bodily symptom experience. In short, they are believed. This is vital to engaging participants because over time, when multiple tests and scans come back negative, indicating that there is nothing physically wrong with their body, when there clearly is something wrong, they feel that they are no longer believed.

Greater connection and attunement to the self is facilitated in TBMA and this encourages self-regulation and agency (see Chapter 1). This is important as it leads to empowerment of the individual to take back control of their life as opposed to feelings of being out of control or of being controlled by the symptom.

The approach honours the wisdom of the body using the fundamental inter-relationship between body and mind, hence the use of the term "BodyMind" rather than "mind-body". It also recognises the wisdom of the body in terms of its memory of past events and their effects, as well as current ones, in line with the insights of van der Kolk's (2014) *The Body Keeps the Score* in the transformation of trauma and Gabor Maté's (2003) *When the Body Says No* in relation to the cost of hidden stress.

The principle of recovery is used, giving hope to people to live well with their symptom rather than just having to "learn to live with it", which is the message that many MUS/BDD patients will have already encountered. There is therefore an understanding that each person is different and is supported to make their own choices whilst being listened to and treated with dignity. There is an ethos of working in partnership and collaboration between the participant, facilitator and the group. Self-acceptance and developing a positive and meaningful sense of identity are also promoted.

There is an implicit underlying principle that MUS/BDD have similar aetiology and are therefore amenable to TBMA. Thus, it can be applied to those with a variety of symptoms in the same group, making groups heterogeneous. Indeed, it is often the case that participants suffer more than one symptom. This makes TBMA distinctive and powerful in its delivery to address MUS/BDD.

A Comparison between Cognitive Behaviour Therapy and The BodyMind Approach

Differences

Amongst the psychological therapies in mental health services, cognitive behaviour therapy (CBT) is solely a "talking therapy", with an emphasis on behaviour rather than the unconscious surfaced via spontaneous movement, the arts, symbol, metaphor, embodied experience or emotions. Whilst TBMA is an embodied method stressing experiential learning, it does not omit talking. It works with bodily sensations and the feelings associated with them. A variety of creative, expressive methods are employed to access the symptom and help develop a new understanding of the symptom and its meaning as well as a changed relationship with it.

In helping patients to manage problems, TBMA starts with the experience of the bodily symptom and goes on to use it as a detector of the need for change, whereas CBT helps manage problems by a focus on changing thoughts and behaviour. In mental health services, where CBT is normally delivered individually, it is commonly used for anxiety and depression, other mental and physical problems, and people with the long-term health condition of MUS/BDD. Considerable work in TBMA has focussed on MUS, however, it is likely that it could also be used for other, physical medically explained conditions and mental health concerns.

The mental health label of CBT is often rejected by MUS patients whose experience is physical. The BodyMind Approach is more acceptable and accessible to patients as it starts with the bodily symptom. Additionally mental health/CBT still carries an element of stigma and shame which is not the case for TBMA. Use of the term 'Symptoms or Learning Groups' in TBMA also helps to lessen feelings of stigma and shame and helps increase acceptability. Additionally, TBMA groups take place in community settings designed to be more anonymous than GP surgery/psychological services to avoid the shame and stigma that people may feel associated with attending mental health services.

The basic premise in TBMA is that the body holds knowledge from past experiences and is the gateway to integrating body, mind and spirit, and hence greater knowledge/understanding of the self and behaviour. CBT is based on the concept that thoughts, feelings, physical sensations and actions are interconnected, and that negative thoughts and feelings cause a negative cycle. Whilst CBT focuses on current problems, rather than issues from the past, TBMA allows the participant to choose to go as deeply or as superficially as they wish. In TBMA the group helps influence other participants to change, whilst in CBT the therapist helps the patient work out how to change unhelpful thoughts and behaviours.

Deliveries of TBMA can be made in a much more flexible way relying on the skills and professional training of the facilitator, and is thus able to be responsive to the needs of each group. A CBT programme relies heavily on a rigidly prescribed structure provided in the manual into which the patient has to fit and does not address any wider problems in systems or families that may have a significant impact on someone's health and wellbeing. Whilst TBMA focuses on the symptom it uses a biopsychosocial approach and invites participants to gain personal insight from their experiences within their environmental context. Inevitably this may lead the participant to touch on systemic or family issues. Co-occurring depression and/or anxiety often found in people with MUS/BDD also reduce as a result of TBMA programmes. Finally, CBT is delivered individually in contrast to TBMA where the group is key to changing behaviour.

Both approaches work best if the participant commits to the process and sticks with it. However, accepting CBT means acknowledging that it is a mental health issue, and this is problematic for people suffering MUS/BDD which involves a compelling felt body experience. TBMA is front loaded with sessions which encourage participants to bond with other members of the group and commit to the programme, thus reducing the attrition rate.

Similarities

Whilst both CBT and TBMA cannot cure the physical symptoms of MUS/BDD conditions, they both aim to help people cope better with their symptoms. Both CBT and TBMA aim to teach strategies that can be used to self-manage symptoms in everyday life, after the programme has finished. Both can be as effective as medicine and may be helpful in cases where medicine alone has not worked. These two approaches may at times involve confronting emotions and anxieties meaning that participants may experience initial periods where they are anxious or emotionally uncomfortable. At such times in TBMA participants are supported by the facilitator and the group and there are always alternative exercises or practices with which people can engage.

In summary, CBT and TBMA are both modalities that aim to improve mental health and wellbeing, but they differ in their underlying principles, techniques and focus. Here is a summary of the comparisons between the two:

- Their theoretical foundations are very different. CBT is rooted in the behavioural, cognitive model, which posits that our thoughts and behaviours are interconnected, and that changing negative or distorted thoughts can lead to changes in emotions and behaviours.

- In contrast TBMA is associated with humanistic psychology and mindfulness meditation. It integrates Eastern philosophies and practices, emphasising the interconnectedness (bidirectionality) of mind and body. It draws from practices such as authentic movement (Payne, 2025), and body awareness to promote both mental and physical wellbeing and aims to support people with MUS/BDD to self-manage their symptoms.

- In CBT the primary focus is on identifying and changing maladaptive behaviours which it is assumed arise from thoughts, rather than feelings. It aims to alleviate symptoms of various mental health difficulties by teaching individuals to recognise and challenge negative thinking and replace it with more adaptive thoughts and behaviours. It is a top-down model.

- Drawing upon embodied cognition (Thompson & Varela, 2001), TBMA focuses on cultivating present moment awareness, acceptance and compassion toward one's thoughts, emotions and bodily sensations. It emphasises the role of the body in experiencing and processing emotions and encourages individuals to develop a non-judgmental attitude toward their embodied experiences. As Gallagher (2023) states, embodied cognition can include approaches ranging from conservative versions close to standard computational models of the mind to more radical, non-representational accounts.

- Techniques in CBT include cognitive restructuring, behavioural experiments, exposure therapy and problem-solving skills training to help individuals challenge and change their maladaptive thoughts and behaviours.

- In TBMA, embodied active imagination (adaptive authentic movement) mindfulness in motion, body scanning, various arts practices and breathwork help individuals develop greater awareness of their bodily sensations, emotions, and thoughts, as well as cultivate skills for self-regulation and stress reduction. It is a bottom-up model

- Although CBT is widely used for various mental health conditions, including depression, anxiety disorders, obsessive compulsive disorder (OCD), post-traumatic stress disorder (PTSD), and eating disorders it is rarely used for treating people with MUS/BDD. This is mainly because MUS/BDD sufferers refuse any mental health treatment due to the stigma. If they do take up the GP referral, they only stay for one session if they go at all. It is typically delivered by psychologists or wellbeing practitioners in mental health facilities in a structured, time-limited format, often consisting of a set number of individual sessions and tightly manualised, failing to take account of the idiosyncratic nature of people experiencing MUS/BDD.

- Despite being developed for MUS self-management, TBMA could also be applied to common mental health conditions such as anxiety and/or depression since these are co-morbid with MUS/BDD and the research suggested they improve alongside the symptom distress. It can be delivered through structured group programmes with a trained facilitator.

- While CBT primarily focuses on cognitive and behavioural techniques, some therapists may integrate elements of mindfulness or body-centred approaches into their practice, particularly for clients who may benefit from a more holistic approach. However, there is little evidence that this is effective.
- Since TBMA inherently integrates mindfulness and creative, body-centred practices, emphasising the interconnectedness of mind and body throughout the therapeutic process, it is more able to tailor each session to the group rather than rely on a structured manual into which everyone has to fit.
- CBT is delivered individually for six sessions usually. In contract TBMA delivery is in a group setting over a three-month duration, with follow up nudges on action plans for the following six months.

Traditional "in the head" approaches such as CBT have been criticised for the following reasons: (1) neglect of body and emotions; (2) overemphasis on individualistic models, neglecting the impact of social and cultural contexts on mental health; (3) limited effectiveness for trauma and complex issues; and (4) potential for over-intellectualisation and emotional disconnection, leading to a hinderance in processing and healing (Pietrzak et al., 2018).

Many fields, including cognitive psychology, sociology, anthropology and neuroscience (Csordas, 1993; Damasio, 1999; Ignatow, 2007; Lakoff & Johnson, 2008; Varela, Thompson & Rosch, 2017), recognise embodied experience as a necessity for learning, emotional wellbeing, healing and social interaction. Embodiment recognises that sensory inputs and motor outputs are integral to cognitive processes (Payne & Brooks, 2019).

In summary, while both CBT and TBMA aim to improve mental health and wellbeing, they differ in their theoretical foundations, focus, techniques, application, and integration of mindfulness and body-centred practices. In CBT the target is mainly cognitive and behavioural patterns, whereas TBMA emphasises present moment awareness, sensory experience, meaning making from bodily experience and self/body compassion/acceptance of thoughts, emotions and bodily sensations.

An Economic Analysis of The BodyMind Approach

In 2008 funding was received by the University of Hertfordshire and the Eastern Development Agency to conduct a cost benefit analysis of TBMA when compared to CBT. The project was undertaken by Dr R. Fordham, a health economist, who devised the model which can be requested from the authors. The following section is the report which was prepared.

The Brief

The purpose of this report was to assess the extent of the possible savings and costs of using group TBMA to treat MUS that manifest as physical symptoms. The examination of costs is from the NHS perspective (primary and secondary care) only.

The approach taken was to model these costs/savings given both known and unknown data likely to influence the service. A cost model for a population roughly equivalent to the then termed Primary Care Trust (PCT) (thereafter Clinical Commissioning Group and more recently Integrated Care Board) of 200,000 people was used to estimate the extent of potential costs under different assumptions about the cost and savings derived from TBMA. The model, once set up, was deterministic and does not consider variability due to risk or uncertainty (other than by changing parameter estimates in a stepwise manner). The model was evidence based, as far as estimates were available, and built in an Excel Spreadsheet allowing different assumptions to be entered interactively by the user. The results in terms of total savings to the NHS services are automatically calculated.

This model was built from scratch following an appraisal of a model used by GPs that was developed in Suffolk (Hague, 2008). The model is designed solely with MUS patients in mind, specifically those with a MUS/somatoform expression of their symptoms which are likely to cause demand for NHS resources. Treatment is based on TBMA approach to these conditions and is assumed to be as effective as normal management but using different resources, i.e., it is strictly only a cost-minimisation analysis (Drummond et al., 2005). This assumes that treatment is based on TBMA for these conditions and is as effective as normal management. Hence the only relevant economic issue is whether there is a difference in resource use under alternative management. In this respect the University of Hertfordshire has been evaluating the effectiveness to ensure equivalent or better outcomes than GP care in a separate evaluation project.

For the model to be meaningful, an initial set of assumptions that appear realistic are entered. The logic of how patients present and how they are treated was based on evidence as well as expert opinion. Once the logic pathway was created a series of assumptions about values to be used was made. These are the "baseline" assumptions and were derived from available UK data and evidence. Following this, new assumptions can be added iteratively to see what the effect of one or more combined changes in the model's assumptions has on the total costs.

The model was population based and set up to reflect a standard PCT's (now Integrated Care Board/ICB) population of around 200,000 persons (this can be changed as required). A standardised UK population profile was assumed, i.e. that the population under consideration had similar population characteristics in respect to age, gender, ethnicity and prevalence of MUS as the average UK population.

Known parameters in the model were:

- Absolute population (e.g., 200,000)
- Percentage of 16–65-year-olds (the treatment target age range)
- The cost of a GP consultation
- The percentage of MUS patients in the population
- The percentage of MUS patients with somatoform disorder (SD)/MUS
- The average cost of an outpatient consultation (mean of eight selected specialities)

Estimated parameters in the model were:

- Percentage of patients in the population annually who consult their GP
- Average number of annual GP consultations with/without TBMA treatment available
- GP detection rate of MUS (with/without TBMA to identify suitable patients)
- The percentage of patients treatable with TBMA
- The effectiveness ("cure") rate of TBMA (left dormant but to be used once known to develop a cost-effectiveness model)
- The percentage of patients referred to secondary care with/without TBMA care
- The percentage of secondary (inter-specialty) referrals with/without TBMA
- The cost of inter-specialty referrals

Each of the above can be varied to suit local conditions.

Note: The lack of firm data on these unknown parameters could substantially alter the model output and hence further research is still required into some of these estimates.

The Base Model

The baseline assumptions in the model are shown below:

In a typical PCT population of 200,000, approximately 124,000 people are likely to be aged 16–64 years old. Of these, it is assumed that in a year around half (62,000) of them will see their GP (this assumes that every person is registered with a GP which is unlikely to be the case everywhere). In populations with high deprivation scores and/or a greater ethnicity mix, the number of patient consultations is likely to be higher. But this can only be estimated locally using deprivation indices etc. In the base model it is set at 1 (i.e. no difference from the national average).

Of these consultations a limited literature reports that 20% of patients may be MUS related and of these 16% of these patients may have a persistent MUS/somatoform disorder (Nimnuan, Hotopf & Wesseley, 2001). The annual number of GP consultations for such conditions is generally acknowledged to be an above average number of annual consultations for all patients (5.3). However, it has been set only marginally higher in the base model at six visits per annum. This is a very conservative estimate.

It has also been assumed that a longer GP consultation will be utilised by this type of patient (whether treated concurrently with TBMA or not) and hence the higher consultation cost of £50 per visit was used (Curtis, 2008). A shorter consultation cost could be adopted for all patients and although this would reduce total cost it would not change the ratio of consultation costs between TBMA and usual care patients, unless TBMA-treated patients were assumed subsequently to use shorter consultations. Hence keeping the duration of the consultation the same is a conservative assumption in the model.

Of MUS patients it is assumed that 20% would normally be referred to secondary care in the process of investigating physical complaints. This may be a conservative estimate as it is likely that a greater number of patients will require specialist investigation, and a higher proportion will remain in the secondary care system for a considerable time. Similarly, it is assumed that 10% of the referrals to secondary care will be cross-referred to another speciality. Because of the higher cost there is greater potential for savings in secondary care than in primary care (discussed below).

Base Assumptions with TBMA Service in Place

Within a typical PCT (previous term, now termed Integrated Care Boards/ ICB), it is assumed that with an active TBMA service available to GPs and their patients about 992 patients will be identified as potentially in need of this service. However, for various reasons it is assumed (conservatively) that only half (496) of those identified with MUS would actually be willing to be treated. At present the "effectively treated" cell in the model is unused, but it could be activated in future e.g. if a cost per "cured" patient is needed.

The actual cost of a TBMA programme at the time of the analysis was unknown, but a full course has been estimated to be around £370 per patient including fixed set-up costs (if delivered in a group session with a minimum of six people). This is based on the cost of a trained facilitator running the group assumed to be £35 (equivalent fee today would be £50–70.00) per hour. However, this is perhaps at the lower-end of the pay-scale and will vary depending on the grade of the facilitator. This can be recalculated and entered into the model. In the base case it is assumed that if a patient enrols for a full course of TBMA therapy (12x2 hour sessions plus pre and post individual meetings with the facilitator) that this will have the effect of reducing a number of GP consultations from eight to two per year. In the base case it was assumed there would be 50% (or three) fewer GP visits annually.

It was also assumed that referrals to secondary care could be halved by the availability of TBMA (to 10%). But this is an arbitrary estimate as it is uncertain what impact this service will have on secondary referrals as little published evidence exists. In addition, the level of inter-specialty referral is not assumed to change (i.e. remaining at 10% of all secondary admissions).

Results of Base Model

For Primary Care

Using the above assumptions, overall TBMA as an intervention saves in the region of £17,500 in terms of total primary care costs when the above assumptions are made. Apart from the uncertainty of the cost of TBMA, the key determinant appears to be the number of GP consults that would be offset by employing TBMA. In other words, what is saved in GP consultations is made up for by the additional cost of TBMA service (as the model was set this is a ratio of 3:1). However, if there is no change in patient consultations or only a slight change then TBMA management would more than add to the costs of primary care. For example, if consults only fell by two a year (or GP visits of such patients were lower than six per patient a year to begin with) then an additional cost to primary care of £24,800 would be incurred. Or if there is no change to the total number of consults the net cost to primary care of TBMA service would increase by £74,400+. Hence primary care costs are highly sensitive to the number of GP consultations avoided.

For Secondary Care

Based on a saving of £1,657 per case, TBMA is likely to generate much more substantial savings in secondary care than primary care at any level of assumed referral. In the base case it is assumed that half of these costs of secondary referral are avoided, resulting in reduced costs (outpatients and investigations) of £348,588.

In conclusion, with the model set to produce modest impacts on the rate of primary and secondary utilisation, overall NHS savings of around £350,000 might be expected.

Variant Models[1]

Subsequent discussions of the baseline model revealed some potential modifications. These included adding in the fixed costs of TBMA for room hire, administration time etc.) which we estimated to add another £70 per patient. We also changed the length of subsequent GP consultations once patients had been referred to TBMA (see above). It was also considered plausible that there could be drug cost savings made by TBMA and we assumed a highly conservative estimate of £40 per patient per annum would be made.

The opportunity cost' of GP time in seeing MUS patients was also factored in and was based on the potential extra practice income that might be earned through meeting the quality outcomes framework (QoF) targets. It was estimated that a practice might earn on average an extra £120,613 pa from attaining 97% its QoF targets. This equates to £335 per day (assuming a practice is effectively operational 300 days a year). In the baseline model TBMA releases 900 hrs of consultation time per year which could be used to see other patients and earn this additional income. It was estimated that introducing TBMA through an Integrated Care Team (ICT) might equate to an additional 112.5 practice days freed for other patient care (assuming an 8-hour day). The QoF income potentially gained in these extra days therefore equated to £37,688 pa (112.5 x £335).

Obviously, there are many different permutations of the model one could adopt with varying degrees of savings/cost associated. The benefit of the model is that it is able to adapt locally to assess the extent of savings. In fact, one model alone is unlikely to fit all the circumstances of different CCGs, for example, there are naturally going to be variances around the cost of TBMA, the GP detection rate, numbers of patients willing to undergo treatment, the average number of GP consultations prevented and referrals to secondary care, among other factors. These appear key determinants of the total cost to both primary and secondary care.

To assess the robustness of the results we ran the model several times with differing sets of assumptions. For example, comparing 1) high awareness and high engagement with TBMA versus 2) low awareness and low engagement with TBMA (and the cost of TBMA set higher in both). The results of these two scenarios (one optimistic and one pessimistic) are shown below:

Variant 1)
Re-running the model (compared with baseline) with:
Cost of TBMA per patient: £300 (up 100%)
A GP detection rate: 80% (up 30%)
Average decrease in GP consults pa: 5
Results in total savings of £308,908

Variant 2)
Cost of TBMA per patient: £300
GP detection rate: 20% (down 30%)
Average decrease in GP consults pa: 1
Results in total savings of £298,988

It would appear, as the result of this crude sensitivity analysis indicates, that savings made by the intervention are quite robust. Both alternative scenarios produced fairly similar savings. However, the total savings are predominately derived from reduced secondary care costs. However, this aspect of the model was the least well-tested and requires further research.

Even in a more pessimistic scenario, Variant 3) (the same as variant 2) but with only a 5% reduction in secondary care referrals, there is an overall cost saving of £124,694. However, there is an extra cost to primary care of almost £50,000.

Conclusions from the Economic Report

It has been demonstrated that the potential for making health care savings at the then PCT/ICB level through a TBMA service are reasonably large, even when the cost of running such a service is conservatively estimated. However, these estimates should be treated with some caution. There are a number of unknowns that still make the results speculative, and results may vary in different PCTs/ICBs. It is for local decision makers to determine how these results apply to their patients. However, the spreadsheet model is flexible and will allow for other assumptions to be inputted as more information becomes available. The potential for making health care savings through a TBMA service are quite large, even when the cost of running such a service is relatively high (say, within 2/3rds of the cost of a GP per hour). This has also been shown to be a robust conclusion based on running different scenarios in the model.

The key determinant of making TBMA a financial success in primary care will be its cost per patient and whether it can offset an equivalent number of GP consults to allow it to break even. The higher its cost the more effective at reducing the number or length of GP consultations TBMA needs to be. One option might be to increase the size of groups or to run sessions on fewer occasions (whilst assuring that effectiveness does not decline).

The main potential for saving NHS costs is in secondary care where only a small percentage change (for example only a 5% reduction in referrals) can also offset any excess costs of TBMA in primary care. Whilst this appears a potentially redeeming feature, in practice the two types of budgets are not interchangeable, and it would better to ensure that any TBMA service can, as a bare minimum, break even in primary care alone with the added benefits of secondary care occurring as well. Since TBMA is delivered in primary care the worst-case scenario for secondary care is that there is no change in costs of these patients. Finally, the additional QoF income likely to be derived should be investigated further as this is a realistic alternative source of cost offsets.

This exercise has shown that even with relatively modest assumptions (as in the base case) about TBMA, the new service can pay for itself in primary care whilst also realising much larger savings in secondary care.

Summary

This chapter described the background to the development of The BodyMind Approach (TBMA) and provides a section on self-management, and a discussion of its theory, principles, aims and philosophy. The notion of self-management for the MUS/BDD population is explored and the biopsychosocial model is highlighted. The importance of bridging the dualistic approach to health is explored as well as tracking the principles for effective practice with this population. Finally, there is a comparative economic analysis between CBT and TBMA for interventions with MUS patients.

Note

1 These costings were calculated in 2008, they would be far higher now.

References

Bandura, A. (1977). Self-efficacy: toward a unifying theory of behavioral change. *Psychological Review, 84*(2), 191.

Barlow, J. (2001). How to use education as an intervention in osteoarthritis. *Best Practice and Research Clinical Rheumatology, 15*(4), 545–558.

Barlow, J., Wright, C., … and Hainsworth, J. (2002). Self-management approaches for people with chronic conditions: a review. *Patient Education and Counseling, 48*(2), 177–187.

Bjørnnes, A. K., Parry, M., ... and Watt-Watson, J. (2018). Self-management of cardiac pain in women: a meta-summary of the qualitative literature. *Qualitative Health Research*, 28(11), 1769–1787.

Caes, L., Orchard, A., and Christie, D. (2017, December). Connecting the mind–body split: Understanding the relationship between symptoms and emotional well-being in chronic pain and functional gastrointestinal disorders. *Healthcare*, 5(4), 93.

Calsius, J., De Bie, J ... and Meesen, R. (2016). Touching the Lived Body in Patients with Medically Unexplained Symptoms. How an Integration of Hands-on Bodywork and Body Awareness in Psychotherapy May Help People with Alexithymia. *Frontiers in Psychology*, 7 https://doi.org/10.3389/fpsyg.2016.00253

Challis, D., Hughes, J., ... and Stewart, K. (2010). Self-care and Case Management in Long-term Conditions: The Effective Management of Critical Interfaces. *Report for the National Institute for Health Research Service Delivery and Organisation Programme* SDO Project (08/1715/201).

Clement, Y. N., Williams, A. F., ... and Seaforth, C. E. (2005). A gap between acceptance and knowledge of herbal remedies by physicians: The need for educational intervention. *BMC Complement. Altern. Med.*, 5(20). https://doi.org/10.1186/1472-6882-5-20

Csordas, T. J. (1993). Somatic modes of attention. *Cultural Anthropology*, 8(2), 135–156.

Curtis L. (2008) *The Unit Costs of Health and Social Care. Personal Social Services Research Unit (PSSRU)*. University of Kent, Canterbury.

Damasio, A. R. (1999). *The Feeling of What Happens: Body and Emotion in the Making of Consciousness*. Houghton Mifflin Harcourt.

Damasio, A. R. (2006). *Descartes' Error*. Random House.

Drummond, M. F., Sculpher, M. J. ... and Stoddart, G. L. (2005). *Methods for the Economic Evaluation of Health Care Programmes*. Third edition. Oxford University Press.

Duncan, G. (2000). Mind-body dualism and the biopsychosocial model of pain: what did Descartes really say? *The Journal of Medicine and Philosophy*, 25(4), 485–513.

Engel, G. L. (1977). The need for a new medical model: a challenge for biomedicine. *Science*, 196(4286), 129–136.

Farre, A., and Rapley, T. (2017). The new old (and old new) medical model: four decades navigating the biomedical and psychosocial understandings of health and illness. *Healthcare*, 5(4), 88.

Gallagher, S. (2023). *Embodied and Enactive Approaches to Cognition*. University of Cambridge Press.

Gibson, G. P., Ram, F. S. F., and Powell, H. (2003). Asthma Education. *Respiratory Medicine,* 97(9), 1036–1044. https://doi.org/10.1016/S0954-6111(03)00134-3

Geraghty, K. J., and Blease, C. (2019). Myalgic encephalomyelitis/chronic fatigue syndrome and the biopsychosocial model: a review of patient harm and distress in the medical encounter. *Disability and Rehabilitation*, 41(25), 3092–3102.

Geraghty, K. J., and Esmail, A. (2016). Chronic fatigue syndrome: is the biopsychosocial model responsible for patient dissatisfaction and harm? *British Journal of General Practice*, 66(649), 437–438.

Hague, J. (2008). Personal correspondence with authors. August.

Houwen, J., Lucassen, P. L. B. ..., and Tim, C. O. (2017). Medically unexplained symptoms: the person, the symptoms, and the dialogue. *Family Practice*, 34(2), 245–251, https://doi-org.ezproxy.herts.ac.uk/10.1093/fampra/cmw132

Howman, M., Walters, K., Rosenthal, J. and Buszewicz, M. (2016). "You kind of want to fix it don't you?" Exploring general practice trainees' experiences of managing patients with medically unexplained symptoms. *BMC Med. Educ.* 16, 27. https://doi.org/10.1186/s12909-015-0523-y

Ignatow, G. (2007). Theories of embodied knowledge: New directions for cultural and cognitive sociology? *Journal for the Theory of Social Behaviour*, 37(2), 115–135.

Johnson, M. (2007). *The Meaning of the Body. Aesthetics of Human Understanding.* The University of Chicago Press.

Lakoff, G., and Johnson, M. (2008). *Metaphors We Live By.* University of Chicago Press.

Lu, C. H., Tang, S. T., …, and Wang, P. X. (2015). Community-based interventions in hypertensive patients: a comparison of three health education strategies. *BMC Public Health*, 15(33). https://doi.org/10.1186/s12889-015-1401-6

Maté, G. (2003). *When the Body Says No: The Cost of Hidden Stress.* Vintage.

Mehling, W. E., Wrubel, J., … and Stewart, A. L. (2011). Body awareness: a phenomenological inquiry into the common ground of mind-body therapies. *Philosophy, Ethics, and Humanities in Medicine*, 6, 1–12.

Meyer, D., Leventhal, H., and Gutmann, M. (1985). Common-sense models of illness: the example of hypertension. *Health psychology: Official Journal of the Division of Health Psychology, American Psychological Association*, 4(2), 115–135. https://doi.org/10.1037//0278-6133.4.2.115

Miller, W. L., and Crabtree, B. F. (2005). Healing landscapes: patients, relationships, and creating optimal healing places. *Journal of Alternative and Complementary Medicine*, 11(supplement 1), s-41.

Morone, N. E., Greco, C. M., and Weiner, D. K. (2008). Mindfulness meditation for the treatment of chronic low back pain in older adults: a randomized controlled pilot study. *Pain, 134*(3), 310–319.

Nimnuan C., Hotopf, M. and Wessley, S. (2001) Medically unexplained symptoms: an epidemiological study in seven specialities. *Journal of Psychosomatic Research*, 51, 361–367.

Norris, S. L., Engelgau, M. M., and Venkat Narayan, K. M. (2001). Effectiveness of self-management training in type 2 diabetes: a systematic review of randomized controlled trials. *Diabetes Care*, 24(3), 561–587.

Panou, D., and Baourda, V. C. (2024). Understanding the experience of clients with psychosomatic symptoms in person-centered therapy. A grounded theory. *Person-Centered and Experiential Psychotherapies*, 1–16. https://doi.org/10.1080/14779757.2024.2360600

Parker, J. (2000). *Structuration.* Open University Press.

Payne, H. (2025) Authentic Movement: A Culmination of Theory, Research and Practice. Routledge.

Payne, H. & Brooks, S (2018) Different Strokes for Different Folks: The BodyMind Approach as a Learning Tool for Patients with Medically Unexplained Symptoms to Self-Manage. *Front. Psychol.* 9:2222. doi: 10.3389/fpsyg.2018.02222

Payne, H., and Brooks, S. D. (2019). Medically unexplained symptoms and attachment theory: The BodyMind Approach®. *Frontiers in Psychology*, 10, 433131.

Payne, H., Roberts, A., and Jarvis, J. (2020). The BodyMind Approach® as transformative learning to promote self-management for patients with medically unexplained symptoms. *Journal of Transformative Education*, 18(2), 114–137. https://doi.org/10.1177/1541344619883892

Pietrzak, T., Lohr, C., Jahn, B., and Hauke, G. (2018). Embodied cognition and the direct induction of affect as a compliment to cognitive behavioural therapy. *Behavioral Sciences*, 8(3), 29.

Porges, S. W. (2022). Polyvagal theory: A science of safety. *Frontiers in Integrative Neuroscience*, 16, 871227.

Pourová, M., Klocek, A., Řiháček, T., and Čevelíček, M. (2020). Therapeutic change mechanisms in adults with medically unexplained physical symptoms: A systematic review. *J. Psychosom. Res.*, 134:110124. doi: 10.1016/j.jpsychores.2020.110124.

Purdy, S. (2010). *Avoiding Hospital Admissions. What Does the Research Evidence Say?* The King's Fund.

Renders, C. M., Valk, G. D., … and Assendelft, W. J. (2001). Interventions to improve the management of diabetes in primary care, outpatient, and community settings: a systematic review. *Diabetes Care*, 24(10), 1821–1833.

Řiháček, T., and Čevelíček, M. (2020). Common therapeutic strategies in psychological treatments for medically unexplained somatic symptoms. *Psychotherapy Research*, 30(4), 532–545. https://doi.org/10.1080/10503307.2019.1645370

Schaefer, C. T. (2008). Integrated review of health literacy interventions. *Orthopaedic Nursing*, 27(5), 302–317.

Shakespeare, T. (2006). *Disability Rights and Wrongs*. Routledge.

Shaw, R., and Bosworth, H. (2012). Short message service (SMS) text messaging as an intervention medium for weight loss: a literature review. *Health Informatics Journal*, 18(4), 235–250.

Swartz, A. L. (2012). Embodied learning and patient education: from nurses' self-awareness to patient self-caring. *New Directions in Adult and Continuing Education*, 134, Summer. doi: 10.1002/ace.20012

Tavakoli, H. R. (2009). A closer evaluation of current methods in psychiatric assessments: a challenge for the biopsychosocial model. *Psychiatry (Edgmont)*, 6(2), 25.

Thompson, E., and Varela, F. J. (2001). Radical embodiment: neural dynamics and consciousness. *Trends in Cognitive Sciences*, 5(10), 418–425.

Town, J. M., Lomax, V., Abbass, A. A., and Hardy, G. (2019). The role of emotion in psychotherapeutic change for medically unexplained symptoms. *Psychotherapy Research*, 29(1), 86–98. https://doi.org/10.1080/10503307.2017.1300353

Trevarthen, C. and Hubley, P. (1978). Secondary intersubjectivity: confidence, confiding and acts of meaning in the first year. In A. Lock (Ed.), *Action, Gesture and Symbol* (pp. 183–230). Academic Press.

Turk, D. C. and Gatchel, R. J., (2008). Criticisms of the biopsychosocial model in spine care: creating and then attacking a straw person. *Spine*, 33(25), 2831–2836.

van der Kolk, B. (2014). *The Body Keeps the Score: Brain, Mind, and Body in the Healing of Trauma*. 3rd edition. Penguin Group.

Varela, F. J., Thompson, E., and Rosch, E. (2017). *The Embodied Mind: Cognitive Science and Human Experience*. MIT Press.

Von Korff, M., Gruman, J., … and Wagner, E. H. (1997). Collaborative management of chronic illness. *Annals of Internal Medicine*, 127(12), 1097–1102. https://doi.org/10.7326/0003-4819-127-12-199712150-00008

Woolf, S. H., Grol, R., … and Grimshaw, J. (1999). Potential benefits, limitations, and harms of clinical guidelines. *BMJ*, 318(7182), 527–530.

Chapter 4

The Programme

Introduction

This chapter should be read in conjunction with Chapter 3 which describes TBMA as a model and Chapter 5 which provides examples of practices suggested for a TBMA programme. This chapter covers the implementation of the TBMA programme with examples of practices. Following the facilitator's intake meeting with the participant the group intervention is delivered – a programme of 12 x 2 hourly sessions once a week, with the first two weeks containing two sessions per week at a dedicated time (morning, afternoon or evening).

As a group intervention TBMA is distinct from other group interventions since it has been designed specifically as a learning experience for supporting people with MUS to self-manage their symptoms. Furthermore, although many practices can be delivered as individual psychotherapy this is not the aim of TBMA which is to support self-management (please refer to Chapter 2 in which further details of the TBMA model are discussed).

The BodyMind Approach programme is delivered by a trained facilitator (and sometimes with an assistant) in accordance with the manual for the programme used in the pilot trial and later refined. The decision to deliver in 12 sessions is based on the context of the wider evidence base. A review of RCTs for somatoform disorders found that psychotherapy treatment in trials was provided with 6–16 sessions (average 12) (Kroenke, 2007). The 12-session duration is derived from research in group psychotherapy (Lambert, 2013). It provides an ideal duration for the group process, enough to allow for depth and commitment and not so long as to overwhelm participants who may be unable to commit to a lengthier programme. Since commitment to all 12 sessions may be difficult for some participants, the option to commit to the first six sessions in advance may be offered together with the opportunity to commit to the final six halfway through the programme. It is emphasised that attendance for at least ten sessions is advisable to gain sufficient experience to benefit from the intervention.

Figure 4.1 below gives an outline of the protocol of The BodyMind Approach programme from early recruitment to the group to six months post group.

DOI: 10.4324/9781003460749-5

Recruitment 3–4 months (posters, flyers, liaison with GP/physiotherapist/pain clinic/alternative health practitioners for referrals).

Application forms – professional and for self-referrals/collection of demographics.

Flag the dates and times to all those referred to TBMA group.

Undertake assessments if desired and then arrange the Individual Intake meeting with facilitator for 30–45 minutes (one week before group begins) to make a relationship, explore goals, ground-rules, reassure fears, respond to queries.

Group commences 2 hours x 12 classes. First two weeks two classes per week. Personal journals distributed. Each week 5–10 minutes set aside before closure for journal completion.

During Week 12, participants compose a letter to their future self about any actions they have learned which will support them going forward.

The week after the last class: attend an exit meeting for 30–45 minutes with facilitator to collaborate with participant to design an action plan based on insights etc. from learning in class and journal. Give an overview of next six months' nudges and to say goodbye. Participant experience form distributed, completed and collected.

Week 6 after end of group: Nudge 1 – text from facilitator "how are you getting on with your action plan?"

Week 12 after end of group: Nudge 2 – email from facilitator "how are you getting on with you action plan?"

Week 18 after end of group: Nudge 3 – self-written letters posted by facilitator to each participant.

Week 24 after end of group: Nudge 4 – tailor-made letter posted from facilitator to each participant reminding them of their action plan and to say a final goodbye.
Next, we delineate the manual for delivering the programme for TBMA.

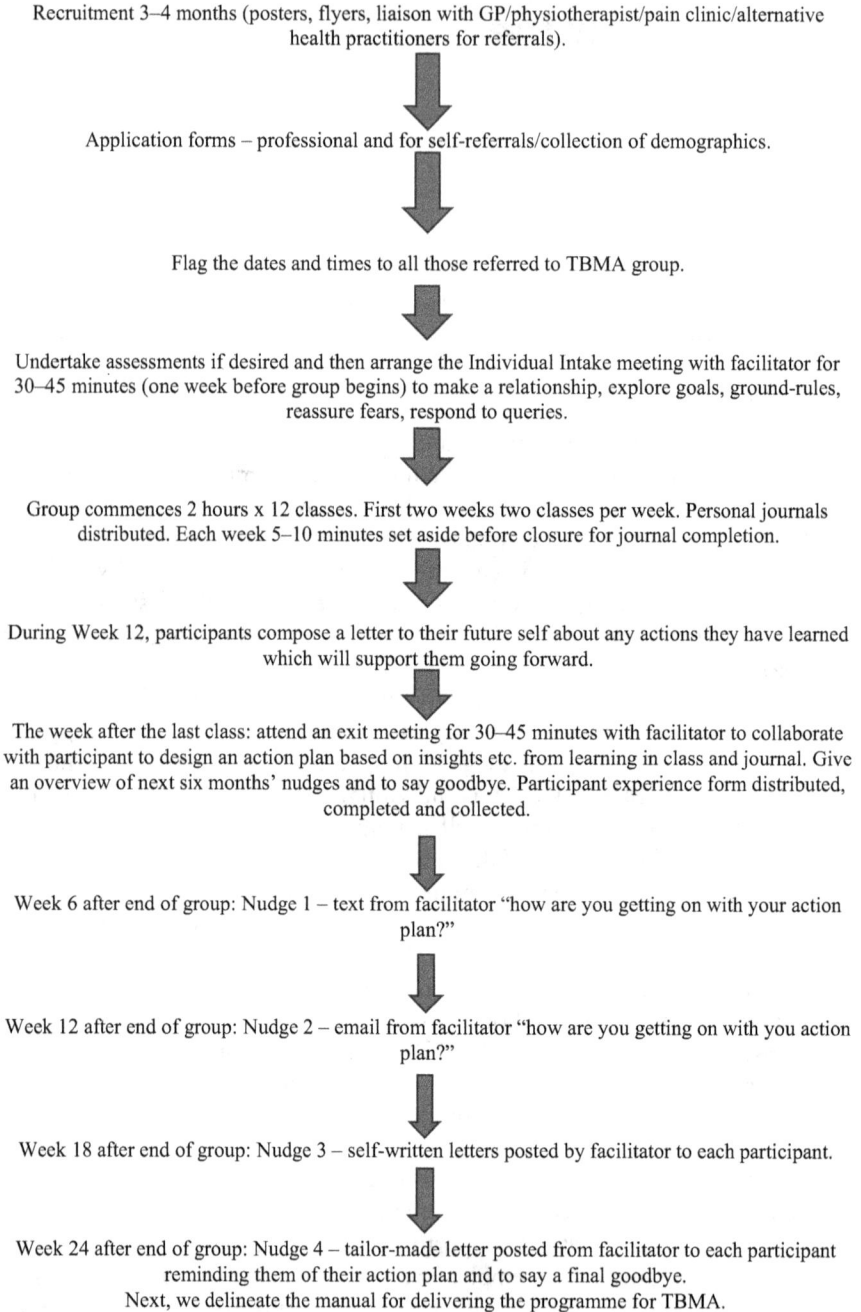

Figure 4.1   Flow chart of TBMA Programme

The Delivery of The BodyMind Approach Programme

The model adopted in TBMA, whilst manualised, allows for highly trained facilitators to use their ability, knowledge and skills etc., to analyse the needs of the group, and for the use of various themes which have been found to be helpful (see Chapter 5). It also values responsiveness to the group needs which is key to cultivating change. In contrast to this, manualised programmes are preferred in the NHS especially to treat mental health, because they are considered to maintain integrity in an evidence-based practice. Manualised programmes can be attractive as research tools but can risk presenting as reductionist and have not been proven to be superior to non-manualised approaches (Truijens, Zühlke-van Hulzen & Vanheule, 2019). Manualised interventions are prescriptive and do not take account of either individual or group needs.

Almost invariably, therapies delivered in trials are based on a manual which describes the treatment model and associated treatment techniques. In this sense, a manual represents best practice for the fully competent therapist – the things that a therapist should be doing to demonstrate adherence to the model and to achieve the best outcomes for the participant. However, because facilitator performance has been monitored and evaluated in a research study (by analysis of practice in relation to participant experience when compared to the analysis of facilitator's process recordings, providing training programmes or video recordings) we know that facilitators have adhered to the approach as described in the research. Therefore, this programme is different from most programme manuals in that, rather than providing a list of exercises or techniques/strategies facilitators should give to participants in a step-by-step recipe, it identifies suggested topics to be covered, key competencies and the attitude of mind in the facilitator. That is, it describes the facilitator's attributes and qualities recounting how to conduct the group as an individual entity (see Training of Facilitators in Chapter 5). All groups are different, and none will have the same experience as another, although common elements of the process can be identified. Therefore, a model which seeks to have all groups into a "one size fits all" is impossible given the complexity of people and groups.

Consequently, this manual is not a guide of "what to do" in an order since all facilitators will already be trained to an advanced level so we can trust they will be responsive to participant need in the present moment. It is, though, a way of being and elucidating the attributes, attitudes and intentions the facilitator needs, and needs to be aware of, when conducting TBMA groups for those with MUS (see Chapter 5). This makes it possible to be reasonably confident that if these topics are covered and the competencies adhered to there should be consistency in applying the 'best practice' across all TBMA groups for a better outcome for participants.

Overall Aim of TBMA

The main aim is to help participants to attribute new meaning to their symptoms, i.e. turning bodily symptoms into meaningful information about their current emotional state and symptoms. Recognising these meanings, participants are guided to inform themselves of their needs and how to self-manage their symptoms in the future.

The group intervention is an experiential, process-oriented, learning intervention aiming to facilitate a more integrated understanding of the participant's medically unexplained bodily symptoms. The approach honours the legitimacy of the participant's physical symptoms identifying psychological and social factors needed for preparing for change in the knowledge they are always in recovery. The BodyMind notion is consistent with, and supported by, neurobiological models which draw on central nervous system mechanisms to explain MUS (Gallese, 2005; Cozolino, 2002).

The intervention relies on empathy and meaning making through symbolic expression from somatic awareness and tracking the body's natural, spontaneous movement with an inward focus, sometimes with half closed/closed eyes. The group is used to promote change in symptom perception, coping styles, illness and wellness beliefs, medication dependence and personal dynamics necessary to achieve symptom reduction and an increase in control. Sometimes psychoeducational input is provided e.g., the stress response, or the way to breathe more fully and why.

With respect to the specific pathology, the "Learning" or "Symptoms" Group offers an advantageous approach whereby the body and the symptom remain the main focus of the work throughout the process. The intervention does not directly address psychological processes involved in bodily experiences, aiming at subtle integration of the somatic and psychological (stress responses) aspects of bodily sensations over time.

It is the body-mind inter-relationship which forms the basis of the learning experience for the group. Stress can affect this inter-relationship, and a split may occur in which the body dys-functionally expresses unintegrated aspects of the psyche instead. Attachment theory (see Chapter 7) offers a coherent developed theory of human emotional development. It proposes that insecure attachment may create deficits in the internalisation of a benign adult, the formation of a robust identity and the consequent capacity to form rewarding, mutually intimate relationships. Collectively these deficits may create a difficulty in self-regulation, resulting in problems in managing feelings, especially anxiety and depression (normally co-morbid for those with chronic MUS). It is speculated that it is this difficulty which leads to the unconscious eruption of bodily symptoms for emotional regulatory purposes. The training elaborates and demonstrates this theoretical base. The approach sees the chronic (more than six months of presentation) symptom as symbolic of dysease whereby the body has to manifest the distress when there is no other avenue.

The theoretical foundation, detailed exploration of TBMA, pilot outcomes and findings are described respectively in Payne (2006, 2009), and Payne and Stott (2010).

Outcome Measures Options for Evidence-Based Practice

If there are to be outcome measurements taken at the measurement points of baseline, post intervention and at 3/6 months follow-up. Three from the following standardised instruments could be considered:

1. PHQ-15 (Kroenke, Spitzer & Williams, 2002) and/or PHQ-9 (Kroenke, Spitzer & Williams, 2001) refers to the Patient Health Questionnaire (somatic symptoms and depression scales, participant completes)
2. W&SA (Mundt et al., 2002) refers to Health of the Nation Outcome Scales, and Ho NOS (Wing et al., 1998) refers to Work and Social Adjustment Scale (clinical psychologist assessor completes)
3. GAD (Spitzer at al., 2006)/GAF (Endicott et al., 1976) (generalised anxiety/global functioning, clinical psychologist completes)
4. MYMOP – Measure Your Own Medical Profile (participant completes a symptom focused, patient generated instrument for measuring subjective experience of distress and the activities this prevents them from undertaking at the time of the test). Shows wellbeing levels (Paterson 1996; Evans et al., 2002)
5. CORE – Clinical Outcome Routine Evaluation (participant assesses anxiety, risk, depression and wellbeing levels) (Barkham et al., 2001) or
6. HADS – Hospital Anxiety and Depression Scale (Bjelland et al., 2002)

All instruments can be administered as the primary outcome criterion.

All attendances/absences at sessions can be monitored for an analysis of participant engagement. A signing-in sheet (see Chapter 5) is provided by the facilitator for the participants to initial their presence each session. Furthermore, the facilitator may complete each participant's Attendance Record (see Chapter 5) on completion of the programme, after the exit meetings. The referring GP/other referrer may receive a copy of the Attendance Record upon agreement with their patient.

Intake/Exit Meetings

Intake meeting

Prior to commencing the group work (the week before and at the venue of group sessions) a 30–45-minute individual intake meeting and consultation is undertaken by the facilitator with the participant. The facilitator needs to:

- Check the participant's contact details are correct on their application form and provide them with their own details.
- Confirm commitment to the 12 (or six with the option to re-commit to final six after the first six) sessions of the programme (attendance at 10/12 sessions is expected so anyone unable to attend the ten at this early stage will need to be excluded as their absence will disrupt the group cohesion and benefits can be negatively impacted).
- Mention a contribution towards travel costs may be offered if ten sessions are completed.
- Provide a copy of dates and times of sessions and venue travel/contact details/address (see Chapter 5)
- Outline the arrangements for apologies for absence (up to two per programme).
- Inform them that 'Symptoms Groups' were developed from research at the University of Hertfordshire and that many participants have found them to be beneficial.
- Outline the TBMA programme and the date for their follow up exit meet and "nudges".
- Give an opportunity for them to ask questions.
- Ensure the two forms are signed and returned: a) Statement of Understanding b) Disclaimer (see Chapter 5).
- Request they speak about their understanding of the group and how they see themselves benefiting.
- Request they consider their goals, assumptions, fears and hopes/expectations.
- Ask them what their bodily symptoms are (and that this remain confidential to you, the facilitator), how long they have experienced these, how they currently manage them, how they affect their day-to-day life (work, relationships, study etc.), date of first onset and what was happening in their life at that time.
- Ask them what they consider their strengths and resources to be at the moment.

- Ask them to describe how they want things to be in as much detail as possible by the end of the group. For example, what will be the differences they will experience and who else will notice these and can they identify one small change they would be able to make to their behaviour? Clarify their goal/s.
- Ask them to provide some history about significant events, their early life and bodily experiences.
- Ask if there are any special needs which may need some differentiation, in case not mentioned on registration form.
- Help them to make some connections between external/internal events/processes and the emergence of the symptoms.
- Provide details on the nature of the group (a copy of the information given to the patient and referrer is available in Chapter 5).
- Clarify the group ground rules and boundaries.
- Think with the participants about their goals for the group, what they want out of it and encourage them to begin to write these down in their journal at this meeting.
- Give them an understanding of what to do if they have any complaints.
- Give them a journal or explain you will provide one, or that they will be making one in the first session, explain you may collect but not read journals, and they will remain confidential to them.
- Ask them where they found out about the group.

Language

Here are some terms to use when speaking about the group sessions to participants at intake meetings. For example:

We will be sitting in chairs or perhaps sometimes lying on a mat; talking and listening with others in pairs; listening to others in a circle; doing walking exercises; exploring what it is like for you to live well with your symptoms; meditative practices; thinking; doing gentle movement, fun activities and creative activities; finding out things together using the imagination; identifying what works for you; writing in a private journal and learning to develop an action plan for the self-management of your symptoms; working on stress reduction and ways to relax/breathe; learning to find support in practical ways; meeting with others with similar experiences to yours; and dedicating time for you!

The facilitator also needs assess the participant's suitability for the group such as age, gender, ethnicity etc., to understand their motivation for the group and to invite questions.

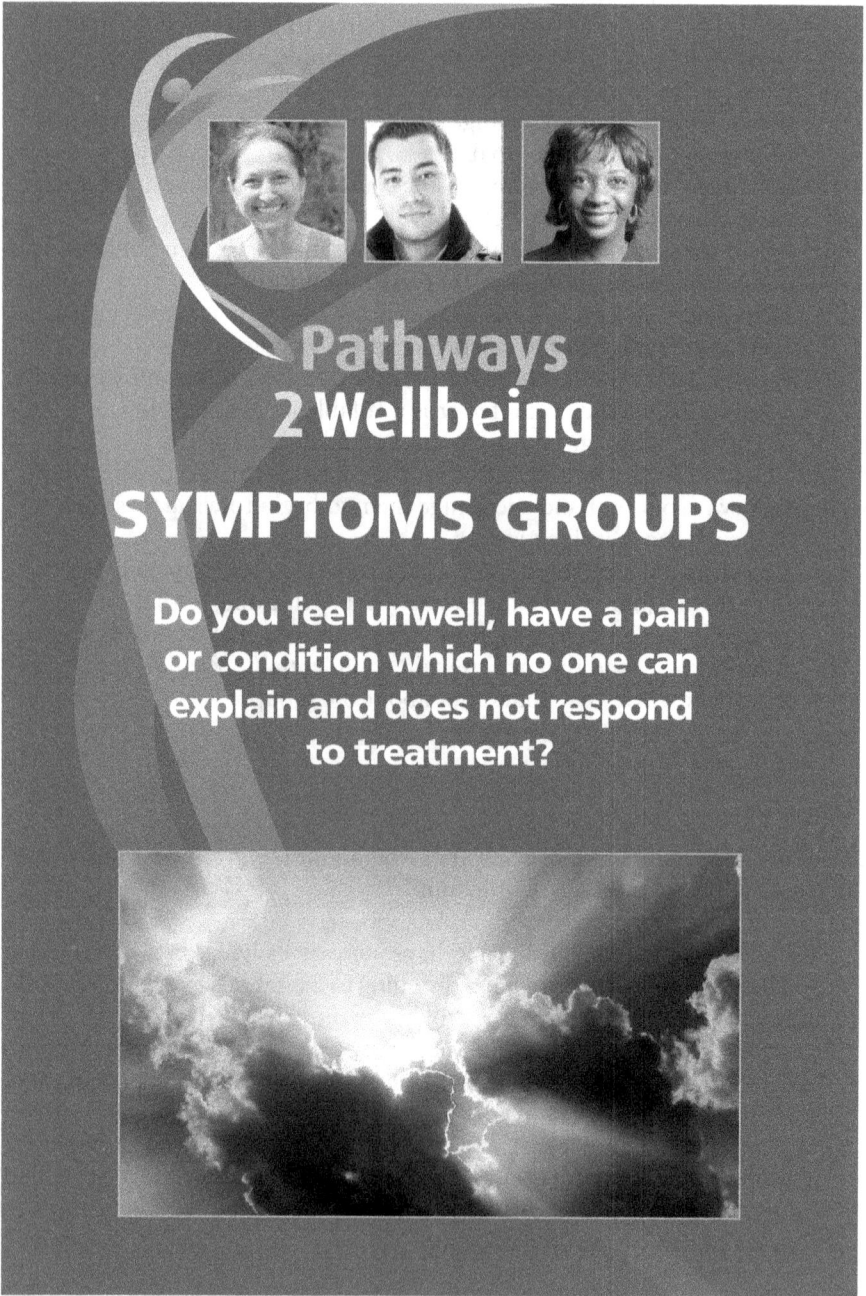

Figure 4.2   Example of Patient Brochure

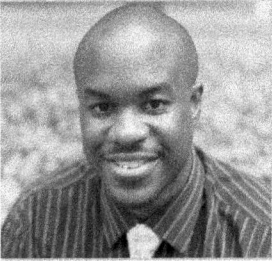

pathways2wellbeing: Symptoms Groups

Do you...

- Think your GP cannot seem to find a solution to your long term physical symptom?

- Have a pain or other physical symptom and no one knows what it is?

- Try everything for your unexplainable symptoms but nothing seems to help?

- Have a physical symptom which is not explained but affects your everyday life?

- Have a physical symptom which is undiagnosed but which affects your relationships or your work?

- Believe your unexplainable physical symptom results in increased stress or you feeling low?

If the answer to any of these questions is YES then the **pathways2wellbeing** group treatment programme could be helpful to you.

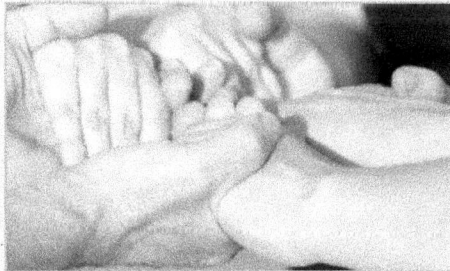

Figure 4.2   (Continued)

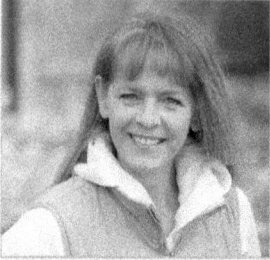

How will the group help me out?

The group will provide a safe and supportive space to explore the physical experience of your symptoms and related difficulties, so that you can gain more control and find new ways to cope.

We cannot guarantee that you will feel better but most people attending similar groups have found the experience very positive, informative and enjoyable and their wellbeing improved.

What will I do in the group?

You cannot do it wrong!
There will be time for gently moving, thinking and talking. Your group leader will encourage you to move, helping you become aware of your body, its limitations and its possibilities. The aim is to help you learn more about your symptoms and to learn about them from another perspective.

An exploration of negative feelings, relationships and lifestyle may be included.

You will not be asked to do anything you do not feel comfortable with, but will learn new ways to manage your condition.

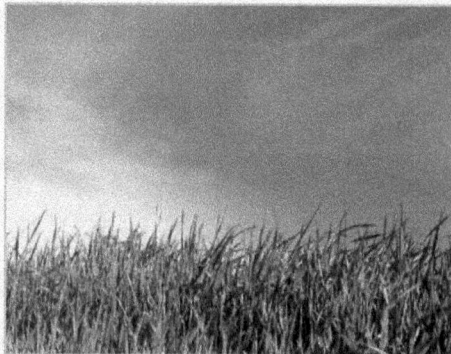

Figure 4.2   (Continued)

When and how often will the group meet?

The group will meet regularly for 2 hours, once a week, for 12 weeks at a local venue.

What else will I be expected to do?

This group aims to help both you, and others in the future, so we will be asking you to complete simple questionnaires at the beginning and end of the 12 weeks and up to 12 months later. If you decide to join the group, we would expect you to stay for the full 12 week programme. However, if you wish to withdraw at any time this will not affect your normal care. Everyone will be invited to keep a private journal to record their experiences, thoughts and reflections each week. Later the content will inform the development of an action plan you design in week 12. This journal is not given to anyone and remains your property.

It sounds good - what do I do next?

Please request a referral from your GP or you can self-refer. You will then be offered an assessment before being invited to meet the facilitator, ask questions and join a group (mornings, afternoons or evenings).

Contact:
Tel:

Email: info@pathways2wellbeing.com
Web: www.pathways2wellbeing.com

Figure 4.2   (Continued)

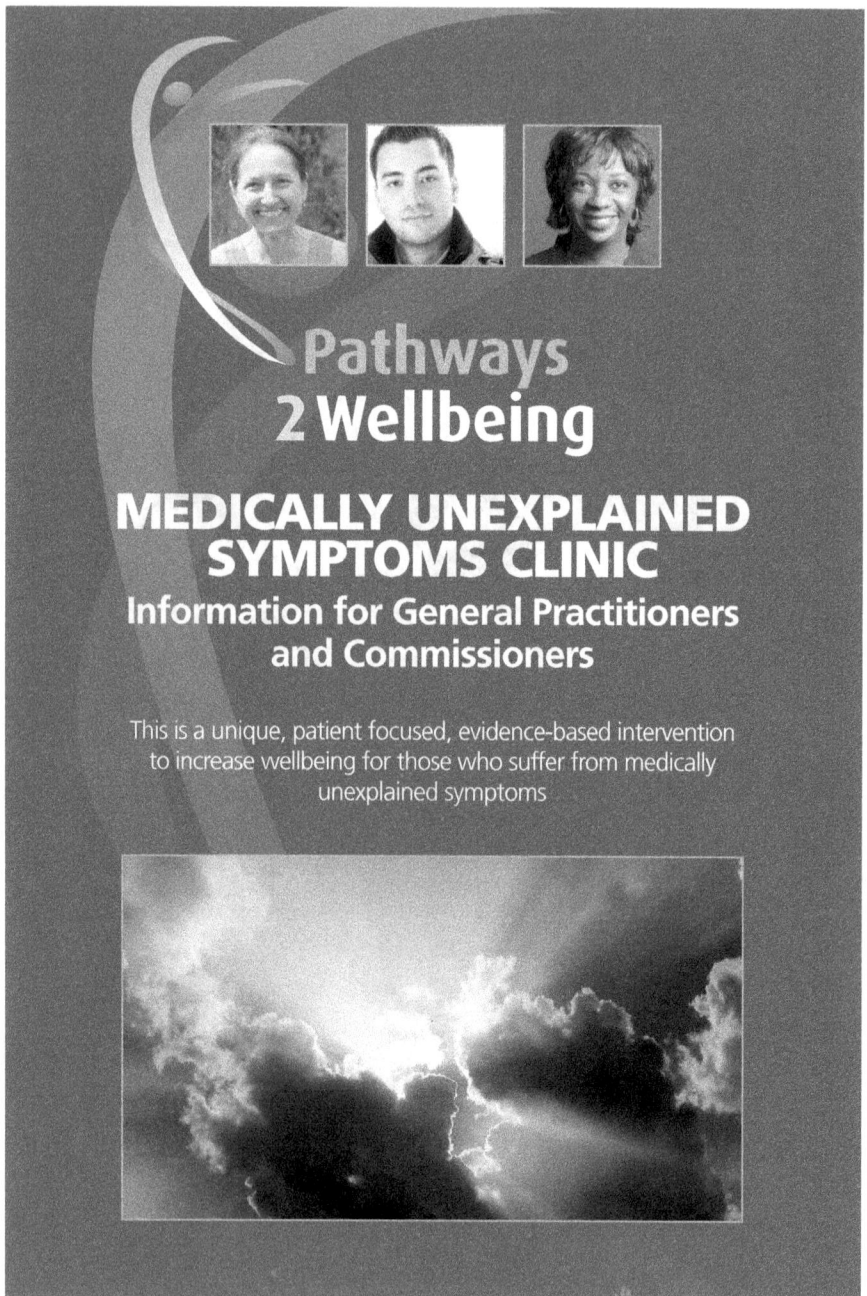

Figure 4.3   Example of GP Brochure

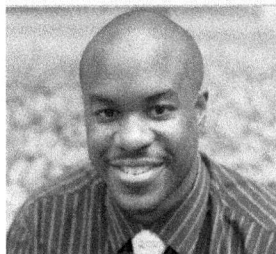

Do you have patients in your practice with chronic (over 6 months) medically unexplained symptoms?

These patients, often experienced by GPs as 'heart sink', are frequent attendees at primary care consultations and require costly secondary care referrals and medication in addition. Many do not access psychological therapies easily.

GPs have told us they would prefer to be able to refer this patient group for support elsewhere in order to free up the consultation time for those patients who can be helped.

An answer to this can be provided by a pathways2wellbeing: Symptoms Group for patients with MUS

This is an innovative approach combining the three major aspects MUS experts claim are effective: a) safeness of environment, b) generic interventions (such as tangible explanations, reassurance and regularly scheduled appointments) and c) a specific intervention. This specific intervention aims to change perceptions of symptoms using the inter-relationship between body and mind, in an experiential learning group framework. This approach has been systematically researched with positive outcomes for patients as well as delivering savings to the NHS. The study showed that the 12x2 hourly treatment programme improved patient wellbeing and activity levels, whilst decreasing levels of anxiety and depression, attendance at GP surgeries and secondary care appointments. Medication usage remained the same or reduced.

By referring patients to this programme you can be confident that symptoms will be honoured and patients encouraged towards self-managed care. The treatment promotes co-constructed ways for patients to control their symptoms by helping them to re-associate positively with their bodies. This allows patients to become more aware of themselves and to understand their symptoms from a new perspective.

Inclusion criteria: frequent attendee; symptoms must be medically unexplained and have been present for more than 6 months; anxiety / depression may be co-morbid; 18 plus years of age; willing to commit to the full treatment programme (including follow up at 6–12 months); fluent English speaker.

Exclusion criteria: diagnosis with a severe psychiatric condition within the previous 12 months; learning disability; related physical disability; eating disorder; complex bereavement within the previous 6 months; substance abuse problems.

Figure 4.3   (Continued)

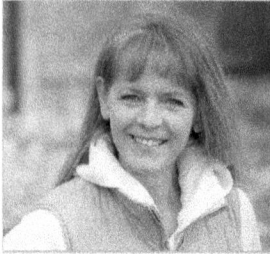

Assessment

Phase One: Following referral an assessment will be undertaken by a qualified clinical psychologist to ensure the patient is suitable for the group approach. Standardised questionnaires will be completed by the patient to assess levels of anxiety/depression and the nature of, and the activities which are affected by, the medically unexplained symptom(s). The patient will be invited to meet the group facilitator to discuss the nature of the group and answer queries. They will receive a morning, afternoon or evening appointment. Following treatment there will be a post group (week 13) meeting with the facilitator, assessment and follow up at 6–12 months.

Phase Two will include texts to mobile phone inquiring how they are and the option of another group either facilitated or self help. It is intended that there will be means-tested grants available for those who cannot afford to fund their attendance (from charitable applications).

Summary

What the service provides for your patients:

- Freed-up GP consultation time for patients with other conditions

- Intervention that leads to patients feeling able to self-manage and no longer being frequent attendees in primary care

- Savings from fewer secondary care referrals and fewer prescribing costs

- A novel approach with proven outcomes in changing self perceptions and relieving w for MUS patients

- Added benefits of positive well-being from being able to manage their MUS and hence having more control of their lives

- An effective service to channel your patients with MUS with proven outcomes

- A self-management solution for your patients

Referrals will be by letter or online through the website where you will be required to register and complete a patient referral form. There are brochures for you to give to patients and further information to download. After referral the patient will need to register online or by post when we will arrange an initial assessment.

Information will be provided to GPs on attendance at appointments and feedback is sought from patient and GP on delivery experience.

Figure 4.3   (Continued)

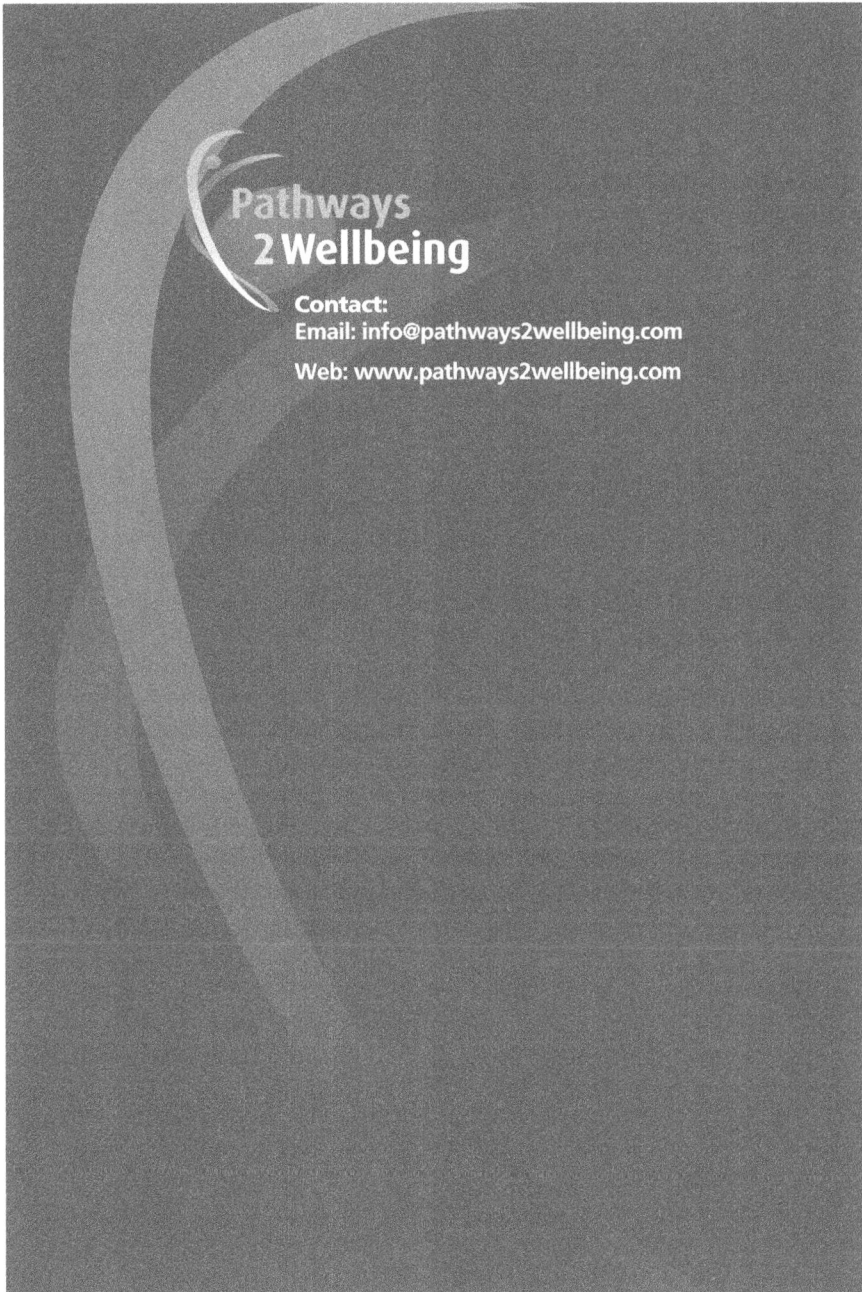

Figure 4.3   (Continued)

Exit Meeting

The meeting should be dialogic, semi-structured, inviting comment about the severity of symptoms, activities they prevent the participant from undertaking. Approximately one week later the group commences.

> At the end of the programme, within one week and at the same venue as the group, another short individual consultation meeting is again undertaken by the facilitator with each group participant called an exit meeting. The aim of this 30–45-minute meeting is to give an opportunity for the participant to evaluate their experience and outcomes further following on from the last group session. They are encouraged to reflect on their goals set at the intake meeting and to make further action plans on changes to lifestyle and any barriers to these using their personal journal as the basis. There is an option to encourage them to complete a "Participant Experience Form" (taking 10–15 minutes) given to them to complete in a waiting area of the venue by the facilitator 15 minutes before or in the exit meeting. Also give participants a "Post-Group Resource List" (see Chapter 5 for an example) on other support available in the national and/or local geographical area (this list is compiled by the facilitator), which can be discussed. Explain about Phase 2 – the nudges every six weeks to help them on embedding their action plan. Finally, it is an opportunity for participants to individually close with the facilitator.
>
> If post-group assessments are to be conducted, they can also take place in a 30-minute slot before the exit meeting.
>
> During Phase 2 of non-face-to-face contact, participants are "nudged" towards embodying their action plan so it becomes an embedded habit. There is a text and then an email each sent by the facilitator at six-week intervals respectively. The self-written letter is sent to participants by the facilitator at 18 weeks post group as another nudge, with the advice they have given to their future self. The final "nudge" from the facilitator in week 24 post-group is a personalised letter in their own words summarising the participant's contribution to the group, their learning and nudging them on their action plan (see Figure 4.1 programme flow chart for the times of all nudges).
>
> Any GP/referrer may need to be sent a discharge letter normally within one month evidencing patient participation (and any absences) in the group and their outcomes from any post-group assessment if undertaken and only if this has been agreed by the patient beforehand.
>
> At six months post group (24 weeks) there is the option of conducting another assessment to check how participants are getting on, which can also be explained to the participant at the intake meeting and reminder given at the exit meeting.

Next there are several examples of the patient and GP brochures for distribution about the programme. Facilitators would need to make their own brochures.

Patient Referral Form for Health Professionals

Inclusion criteria: MUS present for at least six months, frequent attendee (more than five visits per annum), co-morbidity depression/anxiety, fluent English speaker.

Exclusion criteria: Current relevant diagnosed physical health problem/s, fewer than four GP consultations in previous 12 months for MUS, trauma in previous six months, current relevant physical disability, complex bereavement previous six months, learning disability, primary diagnosis of ANY psychiatric condition in previous 12 months (including chronic/clinical anxiety/depression) and/or currently attending secondary care, current substance misuse or in past six months, eating disorder (obesity/anorexia/bulimia).

Example of form for GP/referrer to complete

Patient details NHS Number:

First name   Surname
Date of Birth
Gender: Male, Female, Non-binary, Prefer not to say
Address 1
Address 2
Address 3
Town/City
County
Postcode
Email
Mobile
Date of first presentation
Please confirm MUS/body distress disorder diagnosis ICD-10/11
Symptoms (number and presentation)
Anxiety: Mild/moderate/severe
Depression: Mild/moderate/severe
Frequency of GP consultations
Number of secondary care referrals

Suggested Self-Referral Form for Participant

SYMPTOMS GROUP

SELF REFERRAL BOOKING FORM
Date of Course:

Name   DoB   Email
Address   Post Code

Mobile

We need to know the following information to ensure that you are able to fully benefit from the course. Any queries please do get in touch. Please confirm by writing YES for eligibility after each sentence. If you cannot confirm any one of the items below, please write the reasons and we will contact you for a consultation on the suitability of the course for you.

I confirm:

I am over 18 years:

I do not have a diagnosis of an eating disorder or learning disability:

I am not seeing a psychiatrist or have done in the past 12-months for a psychiatric disorder:

I have not had a substance misuse problem in the past 6 months:

I have at least one symptom for more than 6 months which appears to have no medical explanation:

The symptom has nothing to do with any other diagnosed physical health condition:

I have not experienced trauma or a complex bereavement in the past 6 months:

I am a fluent English speaker:

I agree to contact being made with my GP and vice-versa for confirmation that this referral is appropriate:

GP Name:

Address: Tel:

Signature (typing your name confirms that the above information is true)

Suggested Participant Registration Form

This example of a registration form could be used by facilitators when recruiting patients to a TBMA group. It can be modified as required.

Please note facilitators need to be careful not to fall foul of GDPR regulations. Register as a collector and storer of information with the ICO (for the UK).

(This form can be completed online or manually by the patient upon referral)
CONFIDENTIAL
Name
Address   Post Code
NHS number
Email   Mobile   Landline
Date of birth   Age
Ethnicity
Where did you find out about this programme?
Which GP and practice referred you to this programme?
Please confirm you are a fluent English speaker. Yes / No
Are you aware of anyone else (friend/family) joining the programme?
If yes, please give name and address so we may offer you a place in a different group from them.

Contact details of next of kin in case of emergency whilst you are attending the group.

Their name   Their relationship to you

Their mobile and landline

Thank you for completing this form.

We hope you find the programme helpful and look forward to welcoming you.

(If appropriate this could be added "You will now be contacted for an appointment by the assessor who will provide further details such as dates and times of group sessions").

Suggested Participant Form to Collect Demographics

This is probably more useful to researchers than practitioners, unless the practitioner wishes to collect this form of data as part of a study which has ethical approval. It is not exhaustive, other questions might be added and others omitted.

CONFIDENTIAL (to be completed with the participant by the assessor)
0 Name/ID number   Address   Email   Mobile
0.1 Occupation
1. Employed/unemployed/retired/in education or training
1.1 Employed FT/PT; 1.2 Training FT/PT; 1.3 Unemployed; 1.4. Retired
2. If employed/training absence in last 12 months due to symptoms?
2.1 1–4 months; 2.2 5–9 months; 2.3 10–14 months; 2.4 15–20 months; 2.5 21–28 days; 2.6 1–2 months; 2.7 3–4 months; 2.8 5 months plus
3. How often do you pursue leisure (fitness/social etc) pursuits? Number of sessions per week?
3.1.1 1 x wk; 3.1.2 2 x wk; 3.1.3 3 x wk; 3.1.4 4 plus per wk
Duration per session?
3.2.1 Less than 30 mins; 3.2.2 30–60 mins; 3.2.3 1–2 hours; 3.3.4 2 hours plus
4. What is the support from your family and friends like?
4.1. Good; 4.2 Satisfactory; 4.3 Poor
5. What about your symptoms?
5.1 Intensity: 5.1.1 Mild; 5.1.2 Moderate; 5.1.2 Severe 5.2 Frequency: 5.2.1 Less than once per month; 5.2.2 Once per month; 5.2.3 once per week; 5.2.4 Once per day; 5.2.5 More than once per day; 5.3 Duration: 5.3.1 Less than 1 hour; 5.2.2 1–4 hours; 5.2.3 1 day; 5.2.4 1–4 days; 5.3.5 4 days–1 week; 5.3.6 1–2 weeks; 5.3.7 Over 2 weeks; 5.3.8 All the time

6. Are you currently taking any medication for any physical or psychological conditions?

6.1 No;

6.2 Yes. If yes, please give the name of the medications, including dosage and frequency for each condition.

7. How many GP appointments have you had for this symptom since the group started?

7.1 None; 7.2 1–3; 7.3 4–6; 7.4 6 plus

8. How many secondary care appointments for this symptom have you had in the last 6 months?

8.1 None; 8.2 1–3; 8.3 4–6; 8.4 6 plus

9. Do you believe that the way you think and feel can affect your physical symptoms?

9.1 Strongly believe; 9.2 Somewhat believe; 9.3 Don't know, 9.4 Somewhat disbelieve; 9.5 Strongly disbelieve

10. Do you believe that your physical symptoms can affect the way you think and feel?

10.1 Strongly believe; 10.2 Somewhat believe; 10.3 Don't know; 10.4 Somewhat disbelieve; 10.5 Strongly disbelieve

11. Educational attainment:

11.1 No formal qualifications; 11.2 less than 5 GSCEs; 11.3 more than 5 GCSEs; 11.5 NVQ level 1, 2, 3; 11.6 other; 11.7 A level; 11.8 degree; 11.9 postgraduate

12. Do you have any special needs or physical illness or other limitation that may mean we will need to differentiate and adjust things for you, e.g. difficulties sitting, standing, or walking?

12.1 No 12.2 Yes. If yes, please give details:

13. Do you take medication for your symptoms?

13.1 No 13.2 Yes. If yes, please give treatment and frequency?

14. Do you have any meditation/yoga etc. experience?

14.1 No 14.2 Yes. If so, which, how often and for how long have you been practising?

15. Please confirm that we may send your GP details of attendance and assessment

15.1 Yes 15.2 No

16. Please confirm you are willing to receive details about research participation in the future to assist us in developing the programme for patients 16.1 Yes 16.2 No

Possible qualitative questions:

What are your main reasons for registering on the group?
Please tell us about any current stressors in your life...

Participant Experience Form

As part of the evaluation of The BodyMind Approach programme there is a Participant Experience Form (see Chapter 6) which can be distributed by facilitators to obtain feedback on the service as a whole following the TBMA intervention. This form can be distributed to each participant and completed at or just before the exit meeting or distributed to all participants at the last session. To be completed either online or on paper.

TBMA Programme Content

The following is an example of TBMA programme topic content.

This is an example of Content Over Each of the 12 Sessions

N.B. Remember to make explicit the aims and what people may learn as a result of the experience of each activity.

Session 1

Introductions, ground-rules for safely working together – some developed from the group.

Enhancing participants' motivation and capacity to learn how to manage painful and disabling bodily conditions/symptoms, e.g. through educational information about the relationship between physiological changes and stress for example.

Provide full acknowledgement of their suffering, convey empathy.

Develop initial individual goals for the group experience. What is possible?

The installation of hope, leading toward recovery rather than fixing or getting rid of symptoms. Research on TBMA has shown that many people's symptom-distress is reduced and feeling of wellbeing nurtured.

Session 2

Bodily symptoms and their meaning to the patient. Interpretation is within a historical context.

Registering and differentiating bodily symptoms.

Eliciting and challenging inflexible symptom attributions.

Relationship to health services

Session 3

Drawing out of illness perceptions, stress responses and the impact of negative perceptions.

Education slot – the possible biological, psychological and social factors contributing to the development and maintenance of their bodily distress and in general.

Triggers to the symptom(s) as in a physical re-experiencing.

Session 4

Eliciting negative thoughts and unhelpful habits/behaviours

(Re-)connecting bodily symptoms with emotions, sensations, thoughts and behaviours.

For each patient, identification of perpetuating factors (thoughts, feelings and

habitual behaviours) that contribute to the disabling condition.

Session 5

Distortions in, and the enhancement of, bodily and emotional awareness.

Connection of bodily symptoms to sensation, feelings and behaviours. Meaning making and the consideration of alternative responses to the condition/symptoms.

Session 6

Educative slot – from illness behaviour to wellness/health behaviour (I).

Connection between bodily symptoms, feeling, thoughts and behaviours, and articulating any meaning-making as a result.

Boosting pleasurable sense in the body and in movement action/activities.

Session 7

From illness to health behaviour (II) (for example, restoring sleep, balanced diet and physical exercise/evaluating work status, social network and interpersonal relationships).

Revision and adjustment of initial individual goals.

Session 8

Becoming your own benign friend, relapse prevention and plan for possible relapse.
   Exploring the purpose of symptom.
   Developing an image for the nature of the symptom and its characteristics.
   Experiences involving sound/voice – what sound might the symptom make?

Session 9

Recapitulation of dysfunctional behaviours and identification of alternative ways of being and behaving.
   Adapting lifestyle to improved functioning.
   What if the symptom disappeared? What would be the loss?
   Providing problem-solving skills.

Session 10

How to maintain the learning, skills and coping strategies.
Countdown towards the end.

Session 11

Review of concepts, skills learned and personal journeying.
   Penultimate session - exploring fears, expectation, hopes after ending next session.

Final Week – Session 12

Learning reviewed.
   Action plan and individual goals agreed for the next six months.
   Recapitulation of programme and ritualised group farewell.

Whilst it would be expected for most of this content to be covered over the programme of sessions, there is flexibility session by session dependent on the group needs as assessed by the facilitator. It would be expected that most facilitators would be competent in designing tailor-made embodied and arts-based practices for their groups. This represents the difference between TBMA and a CBT manualised approach, which, though useful for standardising a method for quantitative research, does not allow for people and groups to have different needs. This lack of responsiveness means the CBT approach is one of fitting a square peg into a round hole. This prescriptive nature inhibits the use of professional skills, knowledge and understanding and restricts patient input, engagement and involvement.

There is now an example provided below to give an idea of a typical session.

A Session Example

Please note this is not for carbon copying but to provide you with some examples of scaffolding. Facilitators may build their own ideas of practices groups might need at any specific time and to cover any specific topic.

There follows in this session example a fuller overview of the intervention which falls into five phases, all with gentle transitions from one to the next. It is worth noting that phases two and three are interchangeable depending on the needs and progression of the group. Also, the progression into phases three and four is generally more applicable during the later stages of the group when trust has been established.

Each of the sessions includes a verbal check-in; the introduction and development of structured exercises for individual, dyad as well as group work; and a verbal catch up at the end of each session. Participants are invited to scribe in a personal journal following the movement experiences in each session. Here is an overview of a group session.

N.B. Remember to give the aims for each exercise and what outcomes participants can expect:

- [ ] All sessions begin with participants sitting in chairs in a circle.
- [ ] To begin, welcome participants. Reminders are given of the ground-rules and agreement to them in first few sessions. Absences/reasons.
- [ ] Check-in of how each one is this week.
- [ ] Sensory exercise to attune to our bodies.
- [ ] Icebreaker using the body.
- [ ] Group cohesion exercise.
- [ ] Meet the symptom exercise – whole group.
- [ ] One of the following in pairs/individually or in threes:
    - Explore the symptom exercise (e.g. their relationship to it/perception of it/how to manage it/support with it).
    - Acceptance of the symptom exercise.
    - An exercise to promote the notion of how learning about the symptom happens in the way the body informs the mind.
- [ ] How do you already work within your limitations? Choose one of the following for individual or pair work:

- Exercise to recognise how the body promotes activity towards/ away from the symptom distress and despite the symptom.
- Exercise to honour the resistance the body demonstrates towards certain activities.
- Exercise to discover the relationship of the body as a whole/the part with the symptom to movement (what are the limits and possibilities?).
☐ Activity to facilitate the sharing of experiences as a group as a whole or in smaller groups.
☐ Activity to guide journal writing at the end (10 minutes).
☐ Check-out in turn.

Phases of a Session

Phase One

Building foundations: (N.B. in first session there are introductions, an explanation on the nature/aims of the group and ground-rules are agreed). At the start of the group there is always time for people to arrive and settle. Check-in individually with each participant, exploring their feelings and any leftovers from the previous session perhaps. There may be a brief explanation of any aims/outcomes for the session from the facilitator here – for example around decreasing levels of sensory arousal, the importance of links with imagination etc. The emphasis in this first phase in each session is to ensure trust, safety, group cohesion, verbally engage with individuals and the group and begin to highlight the focus on bodily experience with feeling, thought and imagination.

Phase Two

BodyMind warm up: A thorough embodied warm up follows, focusing on surfaces, skin, joints, muscles and ways of moving using shared leadership techniques and games. Language, music and props with movement to bridge into bodily focus and to keep contact may be incorporated here. The aim is to further the embodied experience through sensory exercises including breathing, relaxation (such as picturing a place where all needs are met, calm, open – a safe place to return to), self-massage and linking the self with proprioceptive/kinaesthetic (bodily) sensations and the other senses with movement, symptoms and the imagination. It is also key at this stage to try to develop a sense of fun and trust, perhaps through a trust game. Breath work and relaxation is almost always used in phase one or two. Participants are invited to enter into body sensing and guided/own imagery in order to learn from the experience and find some skills in monitoring and influencing states of stress and relaxation (self-regulation) in relation to emotional wellbeing. It is helpful to graduate the transition into any internal reflection such as relaxation or guided/free form imagery. These graduated transitions (which may remain) can help honour what is manageable for an individual and helps foster self-care and responsibility. This can look like, for example, participants keeping eyes half open whilst focusing inward, or choosing an active, stretch-release type relaxation instead of having to tolerate eyes closed and stillness.

Phase Three

Developing the theme: This phase fosters the earlier work by deepening and broadening the experience of a more focused connection between inner and outer worlds with the metaphors arising from the bodily experiences. Mindfulness experiences: for example, close eyes and feel sense of cold/ heat, body scan for tension, get comfortable. Usually, participants take the role of the one who experiences mindful movement in one part of the body, for example, and the facilitator (or other participants) the role of witness (noticing any impact on them in the presence of seeing that action, in this phase. As a result, an embodied realisation may be made between the self, previous emotional stresses, current lifestyle and expression of metaphors generated. Themes for the group and individuals emerge, the facilitator using her own bodily experience and group inter-subjectivity to draw out personal learning for participants. Participants are invited to explore ways of learning about themselves and their symptoms. This can be through conscious learning and experiential learning, always connecting the worlds of inner and outer experience through the body, natural body language, expressive movement and the creativity of imagination. All the approaches used in the group relate to the symptom, linking how it could be managed, related to, understood and held as an experience. An example of how this phase could look would be using movement or inner journeying experiences and then reflecting on these through image-making (or diagrams), clay-work or writing. Alternatively mark-making on paper can be directly linked with the body, the senses and feelings by, for example, participants drawing around each other's bodies on large paper and decorating their own image in relation to positions and qualities of sensation and feeling. Group themes, feelings and dynamics are embodied symbolically in the work. For example, themes such as resistance, support and trust can be put into movement with a partner, as can how we believe we are seen, how we feel we are seen and what is actually seen by others (including any witnesses) in relation to self and the symptom. This can be done through participants adopting either the role of witness or mover and having time for transition and reflection. Often these roles can be creatively weaved in as a way of entering into mindfulness experiences whereby the present moment is honoured.

Phase Four

Deepening the theme: Here the participants are encouraged to reflect on their experiences and to share in the group verbally. Time is taken for participants to write in their personal learning journals if desired. The preparation for ending the session is made. There is an emphasis on creating an environment where participants can reflect and be supported in finding and valuing what they know helps and supports them already, for example identifying helpers/inner guides in imagery or discussing coping strategies (emotional, spiritual, social, physical). There is also a focus on finding personal resources and developing responsibility.

Phase Five

Closure: A verbal catch-up always closes the session (check-out). Maybe add a concluding exercise as well. Any dates to note (e.g. change/break) and the number of the next session.

Summary

This chapter offered a full description on TBMA as a group intervention. The programme administration was described including an overview for delivery. There were examples of self- and health professional referral forms for reference together with the inclusion and exclusion criteria for the selection for participants derived from previous research in the area. Intake and exit individual meetings were explained. There was an example of programme content for each of the 12 sessions, a session example and an overview of the five phases of a session.

References

Barkham, M., Margison, F., ... and McGrath, G. (2001). Service profiling and outcomes benchmarking using the CORE-OM: Toward practice-based evidence in the psychological therapies. *Journal of Consulting and Clinical Psychology*, 69(2), 184.

Bjelland, I., Dahl, A. A., Haug, T. T., and Neckelmann, D. (2002). The validity of the Hospital Anxiety and Depression Scale: an updated literature review. *Journal of Psychosomatic Research*, 52(2), 69–77.

Cozolino, L. J. (2002). *The Neuroscience of Psychotherapy: Building and Rebuilding the Human Brain* (Norton series on interpersonal neurobiology). W. W. Norton and Company.

Endicott, J., Spitzer, R. L., ... and Cohen, J. (1976). The global assessment scale. A procedure for measuring overall severity of psychiatric disturbance. *Arch. Gen. Psychiatry*. Jun; 33(6), 766–771. doi: 10.1001/archpsyc.1976.01770060086012. PMID: 938196.

Evans, C., Connell, J., ... and Audin, K. (2002). Towards a standardised brief outcome measure: Psychometric properties and utility of the CORE–OM. *The British
Journal of Psychiatry*, *180*(1), 51–60.

Gallese, V. (2005). Embodied simulation: From neurons to phenomenal experience.
Phenomenology and the Cognitive Sciences, 4, 23–48.

Kroenke, K. (2007). Efficacy of treatment for somatoform disorders: a review of randomized controlled trials. *Psychosomatic Medicine*, *69*(9), 881–888.

Kroenke, K., Spitzer, R. L. and Williams, J. B. W. (2001). The PhQ-9. *General Internal
Medicine*, 16, 606–613. https://doi.org/10.1046/j.1525-1497.2001.016009606.x

Kroenke, K., Spitzer, R. L. and Williams, J. B. W. (2002). The PHQ-15: Validity of
a New Measure for Evaluating the Severity of Somatic Symptoms. *Psychosomatic
Medicine* 64(2), 258–266.

Lambert, M. J. (2013). The efficacy and effectiveness of psychotherapy. In A. E. Bergin
and S. L. Garfield (Eds), *Handbook of Psychotherapy and Behaviour Change*. John
Wiley and Sons.

Mundt, J. C., Marks, I. M., ... and Greist J. H. (2002). The Work and Social
Adjustment Scale: A simple measure of impairment in functioning. *Br. J. Psychiatry*,
180, 461–464.

Paterson, C. (1996). Measuring outcomes in primary care: a patient generated
measure, MYMOP, compared with the SF-36 health survey. *BMJ*, 312(7037),
1016–1020.

Payne, H. (2009). Pilot study to evaluate Dance Movement Psychotherapy (The
BodyMind Approach) in patients with medically unexplained symptoms: Participant
and facilitator perceptions and a summary discussion. *Body, Movement and Dance
in Psychotherapy*, 4(2), 77–94. https://doi.org/10.1080/17432970902918008

Payne, H. (2006). The body as container and expresser: Authentic Movement groups
in the development of wellbeing in our bodymindspirit. In: J. Corrigall, H. Payne
and H. Wilkinson (Eds), *About a Body: Working with the Embodied Mind in
Psychotherapy* (pp. 162–180). Routledge.

Payne, H., and Stott, D. (2010). Change in the moving bodymind: quantitative results
from a pilot study on the use of the BodyMind approach (BMA) to psychotherapeutic group work with patients with medically unexplained symptoms (MUSs).
Counselling and Psychotherapy Research, 10(4), 295–306.

Spitzer, R. L., Kroenke, K., ... and Löwe, B. (2006). A brief measure for assessing
generalized anxiety disorder the GAD-7. *Arch. Intern. Med.*, 166, 1092–1097.
doi: 10.1001/archinte.166.10.1092.

Truijens, F., Zühlke-van Hulzen, L., and Vanheule S. (2019). To manualize, or not to
manualize: is that still the question? A systematic review of empirical evidence for
manual superiority in psychological treatment. *J. Clin. Psychol.*, Mar; 75(3): 329–
343. doi: 10.1002/jclp.22712. Epub 2018 Oct 28. PMID: 30368808.

Wing, J. K, Beevor, A. S, ... and Burns, A. (1998). Health of the Nation Outcome
Scales (HoNOS). Research and development. *Br. J. Psychiatry*, Jan; 172, 11–18.
doi: 10.1192/bjp.172.1.11. PMID: 9534825.

Chapter 5

Training of Facilitators

Introduction

It is important to appreciate the information provided here is for guidance only and is not prescriptive. Facilitators will need to adapt and tailor-make their sessions and the programme as a whole to their own context, including culture, settings, health service and population ethnicity. The material here is based on the delivery of TBMA within the UK NHS primary care setting in Hertfordshire, England via the Pathways2Wellbeing spin-out from the University of Hertfordshire.

Almost invariably, therapies delivered in trials are based on a manual which describes the treatment model and associated treatment techniques so that the methods tested can be replicated in further trials if required. In this sense, a manual represents best practice for the fully competent therapist – the things that a therapist should be doing in order to demonstrate adherence to the model and to achieve the best outcomes for the participant. However, TBMA facilitator performance has been monitored and evaluated in TBMA research studies (by an analysis of practice in relation to participant experience when compared to the analysis of facilitator's process recordings, and the provision of training programmes or video recordings). Deliveries have had a number of different facilitators, and we know from their session recordings that facilitators have adhered to the approach as described in the research.

Therefore, this "manual" described in this chapter is different from most in that, rather than providing a list of exercises or techniques/strategies facilitators should give to participants in a step-by-step recipe, it identifies topics to be covered, key competencies and the attitude of mind of the facilitator. That is, it describes the facilitator's attributes and qualities recounting how to conduct the group as an individual entity. All groups are different, and none will have the same experience as another, although common elements of the process can be identified.

Consequently, this manual is not a guide of "what to do" in an order since all facilitators are professionals and will already be trained to an advanced level so we can trust they will be responsive to participant need in the present

DOI: 10.4324/9781003460749-6

moment. Facilitation of TBMA is, though, a way of being and elucidating the attributes, attitudes and intentions the facilitator needs, and needs to be aware of, when conducting TBMA groups. This makes it possible to be reasonably confident that if these topics are covered and the competencies adhered to there should be consistency in applying the "best practice" across all groups for a better outcome for participants. This manual therefore communicates the attitude of mind, attributes, skills, knowledge, understanding and intentions the facilitator needs to be aware of, possess and in which she/he needs to be competent. In addition, there are session examples, topics which must be covered somewhere in the programme and illustrations of the more technical aspects of the approach.

Research has shown that it is the therapeutic relationship, rather than solely a particular technique or approach, which facilitates change. Studies also demonstrate the more experienced and more mindful (Grepmair et al., 2007) the therapist, the greater the possibility of engaging the participant in change leading to a positive outcome. Whilst TBMA is not a therapy, the relationship between the facilitator and participants in the group is just as important for behaviour change as are those relationships between group members. Therefore, some findings from studies in the therapeutic relationship are relevant and transferable to TBMA classes. This makes it possible to be reasonably secure that if the attitudes, attributes, skills etc. below are integrated in the facilitator, through previous training, there should be consistency in applying the approach across groups of targeted participants, when fulfilling the inclusion criteria, for a similar outcome. As a result, exercises, practices and interventions can be varied, flexible and responsive to participant/group need rather than working gradually through a manualised, technical mode of operation in each session. Consequently, we are more concerned with "how" to undertake the group facilitation for this population rather than solely "what" to do with participants.

The Facilitation of Groups

Facilitators will have a professional training as dance movement psychotherapists and/or clinical psychologists/counselling psychologists and others suitably qualified and be licensed to practise. Some will also be British Association for Counselling and Psychotherapy registered, United Kingdom Council for Psychotherapy accredited psychotherapists, Professional Standards Authority accredited or Health and Care Professions Council registered. In addition to these professional competencies the following attributes, skills, knowledge, awareness, attitudes, understanding, professional autonomy and accountability are required. These will be seen to have been satisfactorily acquired through a monitoring process undertaken during The BodyMind Approach training programme, an audit of previous professional training received and an evaluation of practice experience.

Attributes

- To have the facility to attune to participants and their experience (and call upon if appropriate) within your own BodyMind responses engendered by the participant's physical action or verbalisation.
- To have the ability to stay with the present moment (Stern, 2004) in feeling, thought, sensory awareness, verbal language and with a mindful attitude (a sense of "presence").
- To possess and be able to communicate kindness, empathy and compassion towards self and others.
- To have the capability to hold the group process and facilitate group cohesiveness.
- To have the capacity to be congruent with Self and its expression.

Professional autonomy and accountability

- To act at all times in an ethical manner in accordance with professional boundaries and responsibilities.
- To be able to assess and select an appropriate venue for the participants.
- To be able to explain the nature, purpose and techniques of the approach to other professionals and participants.
- To be able to delineate and communicate the ground rules of the group to participants and others as necessary.
- To be able to use supervision in the service of the participants.
- To have an understanding of, and be able to undertake, consultation process/assessment.
- To support and supervise any assistant.
- To distinguish between learning groups and psychotherapy and have clear boundaries.

Skills

- Excellent oral and written communication skills.
- To be able to identify and assess health care needs for each participant at the outset of the programme.
- To be able to work with, and manage, an assistant.
- To be able to generate an open attitude to BodyMind unity via psychoeducation.
- To formulate and deliver plans and strategies for meeting the above participant health and wellbeing needs.
- To be able to engender a creative and boundaried environment where safeness of participants and self is paramount.
- To enable participants to take responsibility for their own health and an active part towards self-management/recovery.

- To be able to use a range of creative, natural movement strategies organically in relation to group process and individual need competently and be able to help participants engage sufficiently to work with these.
- To be able to adapt creative styles to best serve the participants, e.g. to use a range of interventions/props/art materials.
- To demonstrate in practice adapted skills from within Authentic Movement and either Dance Movement Psychotherapy or another relevant embodied practice in addition to counselling/psychotherapy.
- To have high level group facilitation skills.
- To be able to identify and use the embodied experience as a witness-facilitator in the service of the group as appropriate.
- To be able to identify participant needs as expressed through the body/expressive movement.
- To be able to communicate verbally and non-verbally and form relationships through words and movement in a culturally sensitive way.
- To be able to critically evaluate and reflect alone and in supervision on the impact of, or response to one's own and other's actions.
- To recognise patterns in the group and/or individuals and bring them to the awareness of others as appropriate.
- To be able to offer interpretations to the group and individuals whilst owning these as and when appropriate.
- To be familiar with one's own non-verbal communication patterns and be skilled in using these to facilitate metaphoric/symbolic expression leading to personal learning.

Awareness and attitudes

- To be aware of one's own bodily symptoms, issues, movement preferences and needs, projections, interpretations and judgments (and to own the latter three).
- To offer an inclusive, anti-oppressive approach to all participants and to encourage the group to work in that way.
- To be aware of any special needs and make reasonable adjustments accordingly.
- To offer clear, concise witnessing appropriately.
- To communicate a nonjudgmental attitude towards participants.
- To offer an attitude of safeness yet respond to conflict and promote challenge/risk-taking as appropriate.
- To provide an attitude of presence in the role of witness/facilitator.
- To demonstrate attitudes which promote learning and self-understanding.
- To be aware of the need to communicate effectively with participants/health professionals and others involved with the delivery of a successful programme.

Knowledge and understanding

- To understand TBMA and the way it works with the relationship to the group to release potential for engaging participants in a journey towards self-management/recovery.
- To understand the use of journaling for participants both in the session and between.
- To have knowledge and understanding of the nature and importance of intake and closure interviews with each participant.
- To appreciate and understand the need for follow up contact methods such as personal text, email and letters.
- To have a thorough understanding of the use of interview for assessment of participants' suitability at intake meetings and know the relevant inclusion/exclusion criteria.
- To understand there are connections between affect, bodily manifestations, imagination and experiences and that MUS, anxiety and depression can be meaningful signals about one's life situation rather than provoking fear/alienation.
- To understand the need to adjust sessions in relation to the participant's understanding of their needs/body.
- To understand the need to establish and sustain a compassionate relationship within a creative and containing environment and how this can promote lasting change for participants.
- To have knowledge and understanding of the use of safe and appropriate touch in interactions.
- To have an understanding of physiological and experiential/anatomical perspectives as they relate to body distress (e.g. pain) personal states, experiences and relational capacities of the participants.
- To have knowledge and understanding of MUS from a practical/experiential and theoretical perspective and in relation to TBMA.
- To understand the notion of threat, shame, hopelessness, lack of control and alienation/disassociation from the body present in many participants.
- To understand the impact of adult attachment theory and be aware of how participants manifest their patterns of relating in the group and to their symptoms.
- To demonstrate knowledge of group dynamics and an in-depth understanding of how to work with these to benefit the whole group.
- To have an understanding and ability to integrate the psychology of movement with therapeutic theory and practice for this MUS population.

Training Curriculum

The training for facilitators in TBMA has been amended from the face-to-face four intensive days delivered since 2012 to just prior to the pandemic in 2020 to an online delivery consisting of four modules each of seven contact hours with additional assignments and presentations attached to each module. The curriculum content is based on the systematic research into the delivery of TBMA. The seven hours contact for each of the four modules is with two tutors, held on two consecutive weekend days (two days of 3.5 hours each). Additionally, there are several home study tasks to complete. The online delivery enables suitable candidates from all over the world to join the training. This enriches the training experienced because of the sharing from different cultures and settings. Trainees have mostly been professionals in dance movement psychotherapy with at least five years working with adults in groups. Others from suitable disciplines/ experience (for example, clinical psychologists; occupational health; counsellors/psychotherapists, other mental health professionals, body psychotherapists) all with a background in working with adults in groups and employing body awareness/expressive movement in therapy also attend. Some attend for their own interest solely.

Each module contains a bodily warm up and from module two onwards individual trainees are invited to share their previously designed warm up with their peer group of trainees. All modules are evaluated from the trainee's perspectives and modified in the light of their feedback. Evaluations have been extremely positive, and many trainees have begun their own TBMA groups as a result. It has been so successful that the UK Association for Dance Movement Psychotherapy supported all modules in 2024, the Australian Association in 2021 and will have the support of the Hong Kong Association in 2025. The learning approach is based on active and experiential learning within which trainees are invited to conduct warm-ups, seminars and other self-study tasks to present to their peer group. This enables new ideas to be brought forward and assessed by peers and the trainers from within the needs of this patient population. Creativity, drawing on the already developed professional skills, and an evolution of the approach are encouraged. There are screen breaks, discursive interaction, breakout dyads, groupwork and synchronous teaching.

Module 1

This is the introductory module. If trainees are unable take the introductory module (one), they can begin with module two. All levels are self-contained and normally if a trainee misses a session/module they can re-take it anywhere in the sequence at a later stage with another cohort. However, they cannot enter the assessment as TBMA facilitator (in module four) without having completed all three previous modules. They can attend module four as a participant for colleagues' assessments, however.

Trainees do not have to take the final assessment for TBMA facilitator status if they are undertaking the course for continuing professional development hours. They receive a certificate of attendance, providing they complete a course evaluation form within five days of the module ending.

Aim of module 1: To introduce participants to the application of TBMA as a way towards self-management for adult clients with chronic medically unexplained bodily symptoms at the primary-community care interface.

Content: Introducing somatic practices; the underpinning theory of TBMA; the evidence-based research, facilitating an opening up to sensory, bodily and emotional experiencing; presentness practices; changing relationship to, and perceptions of, (and exploring), symptoms; and raising the capacity for "living well" with symptoms.

Learning outcomes:

- To improve knowledge, skills and understanding of "presentness".
- To expand the skillset for working with somatic elements of practice.
- To understand how the body and mind inter-relate in these chronic bodily symptoms.
- To have an understanding into how research can generate a treatment model.
- To know the importance of the role of creativity in TBMA, for example, symptom as symbol and metaphor.
- To become familiar with the relevant literature and TBMA research.
- To bridge the gap between psyche and soma by engaging with somatisation through direct experience of the self, beyond words.

Module 2

Aim: To further equip participants in the application of TBMA as a way towards facilitating self-management for adult clients with chronic medically unexplained bodily symptoms at the primary-community care interface.

Content: Ways of knowing from sensory, bodily and emotional experiencing; learning to attend to the body: wellness – symptoms – illness; understanding how emotions affect wellbeing: psychological and physical; developing skills for working with clients who are not psychologically minded; the argument for TBMA; adapted Authentic Movement for the self-management of MUS; using TBMA with individuals and groups; adult insecure attachment and MUS; and attachment applied to the programme.

Learning outcomes:

- To improve knowledge, skills and understanding of TBMA for in-person deliveries.
- To demonstrate through presentation an in-depth understanding of chronic bodily symptoms which are medically unexplained in relation to the practice of TBMA within an attachment framework.

- To increase understanding of the links between emotions and the BodyMind.
- To appreciate more ways of knowing to bridge the gap between psyche/emotions and soma to engage with somatised symptoms through direct experience of the self, beyond words.
- To know methods for engaging with the non-psychologically minded client.
- To be able to identify the principles for making the case for TBMA.

Module 3

Aim: To further consolidate the application of TBMA as a way towards self-management for clients with chronic medically unexplained bodily symptoms at the primary-community care interface.

Content: Conceptual framework for TBMA; neuroscience and TBMA; deepening and changing the relationship to the symptom; GP consultation narrative and leaflet; TBMA as transformative learning; flow chart for the model; patient self-referral form; promoting wellbeing and self-nurture; pain reduction through the Chacian circle. Detail is provided about the short assessment of practice prior to certification to take place in module four.

Learning outcomes:

- To understand the value of presence, witnessing and mindfulness in the context of symptom distress.
- To demonstrate the knowledge of the importance of self-nurture and kindness in self-managed care.
- To understand the perceptions of, and relationship to, symptoms.
- To understand the links between some insecure attachment styles in adults, MUS and the design of the programme.
- To demonstrate knowledge of the links between neuroscience and MUS.
- To appreciate the importance of promoting wellbeing (or living well with symptoms) and the development of self-esteem.

Module 4

This module is comprised mainly of an assessment of practice for each candidate and support for the transition into TBMA delivery in the candidate's settings. Guidelines are provided to enable candidates to understand the assessment tasks. There are two assessment tasks to complete. The first is a plan of a two-hour group session in which several elements need explanation, for example the aims for each practice, and any ground-rules. This plan is sent to the assessors and to a peer for feedback.

The second task is the plan for, and the delivery of, a 10-minute TBMA practice to trainee peers which explores the relationship between body and mind for physical unexplained symptoms. This plan is sent to the assessors for marking and as a context for the grading of the delivery of the practice. Peers are invited to comment on the elements they thought were useful and anything needing improvement in their experience of the practice. These comments are taken into account in the final grading by the tutors. The delivery of the practice needs to demonstrate support for the group during and after the practice. This assessment is required to satisfy the standards and quality required of a TBMA Group Facilitator.

On passing this assessment candidates will be certified as a TBMA group facilitator and contact details added to the University of Hertfordshire website "Pathways2Wellbeing" if they wish.

Pass levels are graded into postgraduate categories: Distinction – Outstanding 80–89, Excellent 70–79; Commendation – Very Good 60–69; Pass – Good/satisfactory 50–59; Fail – marginal fail 40–49, Clear fail 11–39, Little to nothing of merit 0–10.

Criteria for the assessment of Task One and Task Two:

- An understanding of the importance of planning sessions and the adapting of the plan according to the needs of the participants.
- To be able to demonstrate clarity of aim and outcomes for the participants.
- To be capable of articulating the rationale for the method selected.
- To deliver a practice relevant and accessible to people with MUS.
- To provide a demonstration of responsiveness to the group dynamics and process.
- To verbalise reflection in, and on, action.
- To give an understanding of the knowledge base and its application.
- To demonstrate an appropriate attitude of mind suitable for this participant group.
- To consider the style of delivery.
- To consider the ways in which an engagement of group members was elicited.

Aim: To further consolidate and provide opportunities to integrate the application of TBMA as a way towards self-management for clients with chronic medically unexplained bodily symptoms at the primary-community care interface.

Content: Provision of supportive materials and discourse on transitioning TBMA into their health care setting. Assessments in the form of practice and planning sessions appropriate for the MUS client populations derived from presentations from members of the group. Constructive peer and tutor feedback will be provided and criteria for the assessment as a TBMA facilitator given, prior to the assessment taking place. It is promoted as a learning experience. Tutors will then mark the candidate on these criteria and give written feedback on their performance.

Learning outcomes:

- To demonstrate learning from suggestions from colleagues on the practice of TBMA for self-managed care
- To demonstrate constructive and critical analysis and appraisal of presentations from colleagues.
- To give feedback in a sandwich format to colleagues.
- To demonstrate the capacity to receive feedback from colleagues.
- To demonstrate critical reflection on the practice and content for the delivery of TBMA to patients with MUS.
- To demonstrate consideration of strategies to take TBMA into your practice and/or healthcare setting.

The assessments in this module are greatly appreciated as learning experiences by trainees.

At the time of writing more than 100 TBMA group facilitators are practising around the world.

Requirements for Facilitators

- To have completed the TBMA training courses and passed the assessment successfully.
- Ideally to be registered as a psychotherapist with their respective professional associations e.g. ADMP/UKCP/BACP accredited for a minimum of two years and generally to have practised for five years with adult groups.
- To be in on-going supervision for a minimum of 1.5 hours of group/individual supervision per month with an appropriately qualified, registered (or equivalent) supervisor who works within a consistent approach and modality relevant to TBMA.
- To have experience and awareness of the requirements in terms of frame and boundaries in which psycho-educational group work can effectively and safely take place, and an awareness of what might be limitations in a particular professional setting. The applicant will demonstrate their ability to reflect critically and show qualities of warmth, maturity and creativity. They will understand the nature and purpose of group work with a focus on transformation towards self-management.
- To have an awareness of ethics, e.g. boundary issues, including confidentiality, touch etc. in a range of settings and in keeping with best practice.
- To have a capacity to handle complex, unpredictable and specialised situations within the limits of group work.
- To be able to recognise whether patients are suitable for the group and if not to refer them to the appropriate service.

- To adhere to safe practice and best standards of practice in line with the recommendation that clinical work should normally comprise a minimum of four hours per week and not normally exceed a maximum of 22 client contact hours a week or the equivalent, for the best interests of the public.
- To understand and be familiar with TBMA research.
- To be aware of, and take account of, diversity issues, including one's own prejudice, issues relating to ethnicity, gender, sexuality, culture, age, disability and how these may influence the practice of group work.

Facilitator Role and Boundaries

It is important to acknowledge that TBMA is not designed as group psychotherapy, although it may be delivered by psychotherapists and draws on embodied practices such as dance movement psychotherapy in particular, adapted Authentic Movement. It also employs some of the research found in psychotherapy such as duration of sessions, safeness, group dynamics and adult attachment theory. Despite these borrowed elements it is designed to be a perceptual learning experience for people with MUS. It integrates, for example, self-management theory, adult learning theory, agency, transformational and experiential learning. Individuals in these groups are helped to learn from each other whilst being supported by the facilitator.

The facilitator's role is therefore different from that of a group psychotherapist. There is more emphasis on individualised learning outcomes engendered by the understandings from practices. Participants are encouraged to set goals at the outset, and these can be modified and reflected upon during the process and at the end where their action plans are developed. Thus, there is a need for facilitators to recognise the boundary between psychotherapy and TBMA. For instance, to recognise that trauma is not focused upon in TBMA, for example, although if it emerges from a practice this will be acknowledged, and the suggestion made that perhaps entering psychotherapy would be helpful. Undertaking TBMA does not preclude people from also engaging in their own psychotherapy/counselling etc.

The groups are promoted to patients as "Learning Groups", "Learning About Your Symptoms" or "Symptoms Groups". Any other title can be given which aids accessibility and acceptability, rather than TBMA, because that term is less understandable and not transparent to the layperson. To medics, though, the term TBMA can be used as long as an explanation is provided (see GP explanatory sheet below for facilitator reference).

Explanatory Points for Health Professionals on TBMA

The information below is for facilitators to use when speaking about TBMA with referrers such as health professionals.

- The programme is evidence-based, and outcomes which were encouraging for self-management have been measured.
- Group facilitators are qualified mental health professionals to Master's level with at least five years of working with adults in groups.
- The groups use experiential learning methods to promote an understanding of, and learning about, symptoms.
- Participants are encouraged to explore subjective experiences through talking and listening, gentle movement, writing/mark making, body awareness, listening to the body and its signals, mindfulness/relaxation/stress reduction, and symptom control.
- Your patients' attendance record and outcomes may be shared with you if agreed beforehand with the patient.
- Face-to-face contact of 12 x 2 hourly group sessions weekly is the schedule.
- Sessions may be held locally in the morning, afternoon or evening to suit commitments.
- The group will be confidential and safe within a trusting environment.
- Commitment to attend all the sessions is a pre-requisite to being accepted on the programme and will ensure successful outcomes for your patient.
- Your patient may attend an assessment at the beginning, confirming eligibility and to meet their facilitator who will answer any queries and tell them more about the group.
- There will be individual, group and pairs exercises.
- Your patient will not be required to do anything they do not feel comfortable with. The facilitator will be able to assist them in finding an alternative if necessary.
- Your patient is not required to disclose their symptom, but the practices will be relevant to the symptom.
- Follow up sessions are provided if further support is needed.
- The method has been standardised in a manual form and a variety of activities will aim to help them learn about and control their symptoms.
- Every group is different so the facilitator will respond to the group needs as she/he assesses them at the time. The following activities are a selection only.

Explanatory Points for Participants

The information below can be used to speak with patients/participants who may benefit from attendance at a programme.

- The "Group" consists of 12 x 2 hourly sessions weekly.
- Groups may be held locally, in the morning, afternoon or evening to suit commitments.
- The group will be confidential and safe within a trusting environment.

- Groups should comprise those with whom you have no previous relationship.
- Commitment to attend all the sessions is a pre-requisite to being accepted on the programme and will ensure successful outcomes for you and others.
- Participants' attendance records may be shared with your health professional if agreed between you beforehand.
- Participants will need to attend a meeting at the beginning confirming eligibility and to meet the group facilitator who will answer any queries and explain more about the group.
- There will be individual, group and pairs exercises.
- Participants will not be required to do anything they do not feel comfortable with. The facilitator will be able to assist participants in finding an alternative if necessary.
- Participants are not required to disclose their symptom/s, but the practices will be relevant to the symptom/s.
- Follow up sessions may be provided, if further support is needed.
- The method has been standardised in a manual form and a variety of activities will aim to help participants learn about and feel more in control of their symptoms.
- Every group is different so the facilitator will respond to the group needs as she/he assesses them at the time.

The following activities are a selection only.

- Gentle movement, thinking, talking and listening.
- Sensory exercises.
- Social interaction exercises. The relationship between group members and with the facilitator creates a supportive environment. The ethos is non-judgemental, respectful and inclusive.
- Using the imagination in relation to what your symptom may mean and its purpose.
- Encouraging curiosity about your body and how it feels.
- Body awareness practices to learn more about the symptoms and how they are related to your lifestyle.
- How you experience your body will be explored and you will learn new ways to manage your condition.
- Breathing exercises, mindful movement, and an exploration of your symptom, e.g. as a character, animal or object perhaps, or working with creative arts media, e.g. writing, making marks on paper.

Suggested Disclaimer Statement for Participants

Facilitators may use this form to provide an agreement with participants that they understand what their involvement will be about, and their responsibilities to themselves. Provide the following in a form for completion by each participant. The facilitator then retains the form for future reference if necessary.

- I understand that I am about to start a set of practices, some involving gentle movement.
- I understand that they may involve a risk of aggravating any symptom I may have currently.
- I have been advised to seek confirmation from my health professional on the appropriateness of the programme or have decided not to seek further medical advice.
- The risks, benefits and possible side effects of the movement have been explained to me in detail.
- The facilitator will do her/his/their best to structure the sessions with attention to individual need.
- However, I understand that I need to take full responsibility for staying within my physical limitation (either in class or at home).
- I am responsible for informing the facilitator when unable to undertake a practice due to my condition.
- If I am unable to, or think it unwise to, engage in any suggested practice I am under no obligation to engage nor will I hold anyone liable for any injury incurred from the movement.

Please print name: Signature of Participant   Date

Accident/Incident Form

This form can be used to record any incident/accident during the group sessions.
Please write a description of the accident/incident here:

What action has been taken?
Name of Participant   Address
Date of birth   Email   Mobile
Name and contact details of others involved if appropriate:
Date   Facilitator Name

Table 5.1 Example of Local/National Resources for Distributing to Participants Post-Group

It would be good practice for facilitators to design their own list of suitable resources in their location and/or nationally if participants wish to continue their journey. It should be compiled from local resources and distributed by the facilitator at the exit meeting. See example in Table 5.1.

Table 5.1 Example of Local/ National Resources for Distributing to Participants Post-Group

ORGANISATION	SERVICES	LOCATION(S)	WEBSITE	OTHER DETAILS
Carers in Herts	Information/support for carers of people with physical/mental health problems including young carers	Hatfield, Stevenage, WGC areas	www.carersinherts.org.uk/	Free/by donation
Cruse (Bereavement)	Individual counselling	Across Herts	www.cruse.org.uk/	Free or by donation
Herts Action on Disability Counselling/ Advice	Individual counselling for people with disabilities, their careers and family	Accessible sites across Herts	www.hadnet.org.uk	Free service
Herts Area Rape Crisis Sexual Abuse Centre	Counselling female survivors rape/sexual assault/childhood sexual abuse	Hatfield	https://hertsrapecrisis.org.uk/	Free/reduced fee
Hitchin Counselling	Individual counselling	Hitchin	www.hitchincoun-sellingservice.org.uk/	Reduced fee scheme
Mind in Mid Herts Counselling Service	Individual counselling	St Albans, Stevenage	https://www.mindinmidherts.org.uk/support-for-you/other-services/talking-therapies/	

Organisation	Service	Location	Website	Fee
Parent line Plus	Support/information for parents	Across Herts	www.parentlineplus.org.uk	
Relate (relationship issues)	Counselling individuals, couples/families, consultation on talking to children about parental separation	Hatfield, WGC	www.relate.org.uk/centre/london-north-west-hertfordshire-mid-thames-and-bucks	Fees negotiable. Some free counselling
The Counselling Foundation	Individual counselling	Across Herts and Beds	https://counsellingfoundation.org/	Fee based on ability to pay
United Kingdom Council Psychotherapy/BACP	Counselling	UK	www.ukcp.org.uk www.bacp.org.uk	
Women's Helpline Counselling Service	For women who have been/are being sexually, emotionally/physically abused	WGC		Sliding scale, min £5
Young People's Information Centre	Individual counselling 13–25s open-ended, advice/information.	Hatfield	www.youthconnexions-hertfordshire.org	Free service

Explanation for Facilitators Wishing to Contact Health Service Commissioners

For facilitators wishing to make first contact with health service commissioners with a view to a contract for the delivery of The MUS Clinic in their locality the following points of persuasion may be used as a starting point.

- The MUS Clinic is an "invest to save" approach, i.e. the cost of each patient with MUS to the health service (whether GP as the first point of contact or a hospital) is reduced significantly. This is true more so in secondary care (hospital) but to some extent in primary care (GP) as well. For example, the cost of referring for secondary care consultations, scans, blood tests; primary care consultations; medication.
- The MUS Clinic was described by a GP in Hertfordshire as the first port of call for patients with MUS.
- The MUS Clinic can be accessed by those psychologically and non-psychologically minded. The non-psychologically minded tend to resist treatment that alludes to psychological distress.
- Outcomes from the research include reduced symptom distress, anxiety/depression and increases in wellbeing/activity levels and fewer GP/secondary care visits.
- It reduces the risk of, and prevents, unnecessary harmful interventions.
- The MUS Clinic uses an evidence-based intervention termed The BodyMind Approach (TBMA) which is biopsychosocial and focuses on the sensory experience/physical symptom to engage the patient in learning about their symptoms from another perspective and make their own BodyMind connections leading to self-management.
- The MUS Clinic offers programmes, each containing three groups of up to ten patients and no fewer than four per group delivered as 12 x 2 hourly sessions.
- There are individual intake and exit meetings with the facilitator.
- High quality programmes are delivered as Phase 1 by Master's level accredited health professionals trained and certified in TBMA.
- GPs need to be on board for referrals and a champion identified from primary care.
- Commissioners need to start the ball rolling in terms of communicating with GPs about The MUS Clinic treatment package available to their patients.
- Brochures/posters about the groups are made available for patients and GPs (see Chapter 4).
- A screening tool is available for GPs to identify suitable patients for referral to The MUS Clinic.
- There is a need for commitment from the patient to attend all 12 sessions or at least the first six followed by the second six.

- A contribution of £5.00 per session towards travel costs is payable by The MUS Clinic to all patients attending ten or more group sessions, all individual meetings, monitoring appointments and returning a completed Participant Experience Form (see Chapter 4).
- Narrative/explanation is provided for GPs in their consultation with patients at referral (see Chapter 4).
- The MUS Clinic may assess each patient for suitability, anxiety, depression, symptom distress and social capital.
- Assessment at pre, post and follow up is compatible with measures used in Talking Therapies.
- Participant Experience Forms may be distributed post-group to gain feedback from patients.
- Phase 2 is six months. Every six weeks patients are supported via nudges from facilitators such as emails, letters and text messages asking how they are doing on their action plan. Self-help groups and further signposted pathways such as the resources sheet may be distributed for further support if necessary (see Chapter 4 for flow chart of programme).
- Groups take place in local community settings to avoid psychological stigma (see below).
- Patient attendance record (see below) and outcomes may be shared with referral health professional/GPs if previously agreed with patients.

Suggested Criteria for Selecting a Venue for TBMA Group Delivery

All these criteria need to be met to ensure the environment is of the highest quality possible for the group.

Please check each item to confirm. E=Essential D=Desirable

Name of Venue   Address   Post code
Contact person's details: Name   Tel/ Mob   Email
Accessible by bus, train and car E
Car parking/disabled spaces/maximum stay/cost/location? E
Disabled access E
Refreshment facility D
Clean toilets E
Confidential space or could become so (say how) E
Free from disturbance E
Chairs for 13 people E
Chairs suitable for movement E
Clean and tidy D
Empty of furnishings D

Clean, warm floor (enabling participants to wear socks only) E
Yoga mats/blankets/bolsters available for use D
Enough space for 10 participants to lie on floor with space around them E
Do you know where the emergency exits are? E
Do you know the procedures in this venue in case of fire? E
Do you know the first aid person at the venue? E
Do you have a map to give to participants for travel to the venue E
Do you know buses/trains closest to venue to give to participants? E
Is there sufficient parking for all? E
Can the door hold a sign session in progress? E
Have you written confirmation from and/or a copy of venue insurance? E

Suggested Individual Participant Attendance Record

(To send to referrer if agreed with participant.)

Participant Name:　　　Address:　　　DoB:
Course Dates:　　　Location:

Session number:　　　Date of session:
Present (P) /Absent (A)
1
2
3
4
5
6
7
8
9
10
11
12
TOTAL NUMBER OF SESSIONS ATTENDED:
Were more than 10 sessions attended? *Delete as appropriate:
YES* TRAVEL CONTRIBUTION DUE (£5.00 per group session attended to a maximum of £60): £
NO* Travel contribution not payable.

Suggested Participants' Signing-in Sheet

Facilitator's Name:
Place of Group
Dates of Group: From----- To-----

Name	Initial	date	date	date	date	date	date

Each participant to initial for each session they are present.
Facilitator inserts "A" for each absence.
Add more date columns as required

Facilitator's signature: Date:

Example of Schedule of Session Dates/Times to Forward to Each Participant.

Facilitator Name:
Mobile: Email:
Venue:
Travel: Bus number/ train station/car parking

Individual intake meeting with facilitator:

Friday 4 January 2013 – 30 min. pm appointment. You have agreed this time.

Session 1 Monday 7 January 6.30 to 8.30pm
Session 2 Thursday 10 January 6.30 to 8.30pm
Session 3 Monday 14 January 6.30 to 8.30pm
Session 4 Thursday 17 January 6.30 to 8.30pm
Session 5 Thursday 24 January 6.30 to 8.30pm
Session 6 Thursday 31 January 6.30 to 8.30pm (may offer a re-commitment to attend the final six sessions here)
Session 7 Thursday 7 February 6.30 to 8.30pm
Thursday 14 February NO GROUP
Session 8 Thursday 21 February 6.30 to 8 30pm
Session 9 Thursday 28 February 6.30 to 8.30pm
Session 10 Thursday 7 March 6.30 to 8.30pm
Session 11 Thursday 14 March 6.30 to 8.30pm
Session 12 Thursday 21 March 6.30 to 8.30pm

Individual exit meeting facilitator:
Friday 22 March – 30 min. pm appointment TBA

Please arrive ...... minutes before each group session commences, tea/coffee/water available from machine at venue reception. There may be forms to complete.

I look forward to working with you in the group.

Suggested Risk Assessment Protocol

The assessment should have flagged any potential risks resulting in referring the patient back to their GP/referrer. However, if a participant demonstrates behaviour which concerns you, such as the emergence of traumatic events as a pre-occupation or suicidal thoughts being disclosed, please have a confidential discussion with the participant communicating gently that you are concerned for their welfare and therefore you will be referring them to their GP. Make a note in your process recording.

Summary

This chapter has covered the training of TBMA group facilitators. The pre-requisites for candidates training in TBMA, the content of training modules and assessments were provided. Information distributed during the training, the attitude of mind expected of facilitators and guidance on the facilitation of the groups were included. The attributes, skills, knowledge and under-standing of facilitators were itemised. The need for boundaries and the role of the facilitator have been identified and explanatory points for facilitators to give to health professionals and group participants supplied. A suggested disclaimer and a statement of understanding for participants were also given. Both GP/health service commissioners and participant/patient explanations of the programme/groups respectfully were included. Suggested examples of forms for use by the facilitator including a patient self-referral form, an acci-dent and incident form, and an example of an attendance record have been provided. Finally, an example of a local and national resources list which facilitators could give to participants at the end of their TBMA course has been offered.

References

Grepmair, L., Mitterlehner, F., ... and Nickel, M. (2007). Promoting mindfulness in psychotherapists in training influences the treatment results of their patients: a randomized, double-blind, controlled study. *Psychotherapy and Psychosomatics*, 76(6), 332–338.
Stern, D. N. (2004). *The Present Moment in Psychotherapy and Everyday Life* (Norton Series on Interpersonal Neurobiology). W. W. Norton and Company.

Chapter 6

A Qualitative Study of Patients' Views on The BodyMind Approach

(An earlier version of this chapter was first published in *Frontiers in Psychology* [2020] 11:554566).

Introduction

This chapter reports on original, pre-clinical trial qualitative research. It is based on an analysis of the views of patient-participants, with medically unexplained symptoms (MUS), on an embodied arts-based practice, "The BodyMind Approach®" (TBMA). The aims of TBMA are for participants to develop a changed relationship with their MUS and to enable self-management, both unique to TBMA.

Five themes we call key principles were derived from a synthesis of the analysis of data collected from interviews and questionnaires. These principles explain why TBMA, delivered in the English National Health Service (NHS), demonstrates effectiveness in supporting self-management.

The MUS patient population lacks appropriate, accessible and acceptable interventions (Chew-Graham et al., 2017). Physiotherapy (pain management) and/or psychological services (mental health, cognitive behaviour therapy/CBT) are the only choices available. The latter is wholly unacceptable to this population due to their physical experiences in the body, which shapes their explanatory model of their condition as being only physical. Additionally, there is a greater stigma associated with psychological/mental health generally. TBMA brings both physiological and psychological aspects together in one unique intervention. TBMA for people with MUS has had encouraging outcomes and there is evidence of its acceptability for this hard-to-reach population.

Medically Unexplained Symptoms

Previously called 'psychosomatic conditions', MUS (or Somatic Symptom Disorder/Body Distress Disorder) is defined as chronic bodily complaints for which examinations do not show explanatory structural or other specified pathology (Henningsen, Zipfel & Herzog, 2007). For example, chronic fatigue, headache, chronic pain, fibromyalgia, etc. (Fink & Schroder, 2010; Department of Health, 2008). Patients have recurrent or

DOI: 10.4324/9781003460749-7

persistent symptoms, or symptom disorders. Patients with chronic symptoms are extremely common in primary (Steinbrecher et al., 2011; Haller et al., 2015) and secondary care (Nimnuan, Hotopf & Wessely, 2001; Burton et al., 2012), and are a costly (Bermingham et al., 2010) worldwide problem.

Self-Management of Health Conditions

Self-management in health care is defined in different ways, incorporating prevention and decline. It aims to increase the capacity for self-regulation monitoring thoughts, sensations, feelings and behaviours. The impact of self-management groups has the potential to improve health outcomes, such as increases in patient confidence, physical functioning, adherence to treatment/medication and reduction in anxiety (Challis et al., 2010).

Multiple ways of knowing (Miller & Crabtree, 2005) incorporates a range of activities to engage patients in reflection and self-awareness, memories, body awareness, dance, body maps, improving body confidence and sensitivity, thereby enhancing self-care. Body stories of health and illness, and the complex relationship of bodies to life histories and context, is through the art process, rather than solely verbal. As Swartz (2012, p. 21) says when referring to this form of health education "patients challenge their own situated knowledge and transformation becomes possible". New and different practices, such as dancing together, result in assumptions about their body being questioned. Written reflections in participant's journals about their changing body experiences help develop insights and connected knowledge with their own and family/culture and collective knowledge. Through becoming more connected with their bodies they can know the meanings of, and respond more appropriately to, bodily messages of pain etc. For example, not rushing to the GP or A&E but valuing, recognising and regulating emotions, thus benefiting them and those around them. Furthermore, this helps people to be able to distinguish between the feeling of connection and disconnection with self and others.

Purdy (2010) found self-management reduced unplanned hospital admissions for chronic obstructive pulmonary disease and asthma. Bjørnnes, Parry and Leegard (2018) conducted a meta-summary of qualitative research of self-management for women with cardiac pain, which supported an individualised intervention strategy. In TBMA these outcomes promoted the strategy of patient individual goal setting, action planning, managing physical and emotional responses, and social facilitation.

TBMA satisfies the above findings through a facilitated group self-management programme with individual goal setting and action plans for people with MUS. It emphasises multiple ways of knowing, social facilitation and managing physical and emotional responses. Addressing the long-term aim of self-managing symptoms in a sustainable manner reduces the gap between patient needs and funding constraints.

The BodyMind Approach®

The BodyMind Approach® (TBMA) was first researched in 2004 (Payne, 2009a, 2009b; Payne & Stott, 2010) which showed promising outcomes. Further research with larger numbers demonstrated TBMA increased well-being, activity levels and decreased depression, symptom distress and anxiety (Payne & Brooks, 2017). The capital B and M in the term "BodyMind" emerged from 1.5–2 hourly interviews with participants in a previous research study (Payne & Stott, 2010). It emphasises a bottom-up process, although both "body" and "mind" are important to connect. In TBMA the body is primary, so comes first, connected to the mind (which is not solely the brain – Siegal, 2012). It also counter-balances current trends regarding "mind-body" concepts (top down).

TBMA, called "Learning Groups" for patients and GPs, is a biopsychosocial model, i.e. is interdisciplinary and looks at the interconnection between biology, psychology, and socio-environmental factors, all of which play a role in TBMA. It addresses, for example, the stress response (biological), the MUS person's mind-set (psychological), and the social and the body environment (the symptom and the group).

TBMA has been specifically designed to support patients with MUS. It consists of an embodied, enactivist (Gallagher, 2019) model derived from dance movement psychotherapy (Pallaro, 2007; Payne, 2006, 2018) and experimental practices designed to explore the symptom, and any meaning through the media of expressive movement, drama (role play), clay, mark-making and writing. These practices are conducted as large/small groups, in pairs and individually. There is a facilitator, a specialist in dance movement psychotherapy (DMP), adult group work and expressive embodiment models, trained in TBMA, who initiates and co-ordinates the practices and the interactions. A manual for TBMA supports the facilitator with examples of practices, values, attributes, competencies and mind-set. The content of the programme for TBMA is described in detail in Payne, Jarvis and Roberts (2019).

The group in this report is defined as members of the group and their interactions. The group experience is defined as the facilitation and/or content of practices, or both.

Arts Methods in The BodyMind Approach®

The UK All-Party Parliamentary Group on Arts, Health and Wellbeing (formed in 2014) encouraged the use of the arts in health (APPG, 2017). Arts practices are central and integral to TBMA. The methods adopted have been adapted from DMP to suit the MUS population, for example, dancing synchronously together as a group with and without music (Chace, 1975), and authentic movement (Whitehouse, 1999; Adler 2002; Payne,

2006). Music is used as an emotional induction tool accentuating group-expressed movement qualities and emotions or contrasting with them. Group dance, ubiquitous in humans, involving exertive, synchronised, movement to music is employed. Research demonstrates there is a link between exertive, synchronous group movement and elevated pain thresholds, even with low exertion tasks. Synchrony and exertion have independent effects on this measure which suggests endorphins have been released which reduce pain (Tarr, Launey & Dunbar, 2016). It may also play a role in social bonding within the group setting. A mixed methods study of group DMP by Shim et al. (2017) aimed to test and refine a model of DMP for pain resilience. It found improved resilience; less kinesiophobia (fear of movement frequently found in people suffering MUS); increased body awareness; reduced pain intensity and stress; and increased relaxation. In the study, 68% of people felt "moderately to a great deal better" post-intervention. Key mechanisms were activating self-agency, connecting to self and others, enhancing emotional intelligence and reframing. These results have helped to inform the model of TBMA for pain reduction in people with MUS (since many symptoms involve unexplained pain).

Another element borrowed from DMP is mirroring (Eberhard-Kaechele, 2019) which has been shown to foster secure attachment, synchrony and emotional regulation. Mirroring can become synchronous (Vicaria & Dickens, 2016). Rennung and Göritz (2016) defined this interpersonal synchrony as instances when the movements or sensations of two or more people overlap in time. Studies on interpersonal synchrony using manipulated synchronised movement show it has positive, especially prosocial, outcomes (Rabinowitch & Meltzoff, 2017). Mirroring promotes dyadic resonance, shapes secure attachment experiences and facilitates integration (Beebe & Lachmann, 1998). Nonverbal components give rise to right-to-right hemisphere resonance affecting attachment relationships, regulation and emotional processing (Schore, 2003). This process of mutual adaptation in mirroring and Chacian group movement (Chace, 1975), can be described as motion co-regulation for the purpose of creating synchrony (Hart et al., 2014). According to Fogel (1993) co-regulation is an intrinsic element of dyadic interactions. There are two modes of emotional self-regulation: interactive and auto regulation. Mirroring and group synchronous movement supports the former. These findings inform TBMA.

It appears insecure attachment is frequently found in people with MUS (Adshead & Guthrie, 2015). TBMA has been designed to take account of the adult insecure attachment styles (Payne & Brooks, 2019). Attachment is fundamentally a regulatory theory (Fonagy & Target, 2002). Secure attachment involves the capacity to shift between two modes of emotional regulation, depending on context (Schore & Schore, 2006). Group or dyadic practices using expressive movement provide regulatory opportunities for this adaption between the two modes.

The rationale for including mark-making on paper, clay sculpting, painting with fingers/non-writing hand, and journal writing is that they cultivate a non-threatening environment, there being no right or wrong answers, and are inclusive. They stimulate creativity, offering symbolic representation of the symptom, thereby encouraging a change in the perception of it, and the participants' relationship to it, to make meaning. Verbal and nonverbal symbolisation narration evolves. This is an experiential means of shifting from a harsh internal mind-set/critic which monitors the threat response, to an internal, benign, self-caring, mind-set, and the associated role that compassion (body and self) has on emotional regulation, and threat management. From the symptom feeling like the "enemy" to be "got rid of", it can change to becoming an "ally" and to be "accepted". People begin to recognise it is their perception of their symptom which is mediating their bodily experience and by relating to it differently, they are more able to see ways of managing it. As a result, there is a change in the perception of mind-set, self and agency. The symptom symbolised by movement, marks on paper etc., becomes the gateway to self-development and self-management. Arts practices are an ideal vehicle for distancing the symptom from the person, making it safer for exploration.

TBMA with its integrated arts bias involves the social model of health where improvements in social inclusion and cohesion are important indicators. This contrasts with the medical model, employed by pain management and CBT which separates body from mind. Additionally, CBT uses solely verbal methods. TBMA contrasts with other body-oriented models (Rohricht et al., 2019) since TBMA, although also working with the body, works with expression through movement and the arts, and has the goal of self-management rather than cure.

TBMA integrates the body and its sensations with movement and the arts to inspire somatic, cognitive, social, imaginative and emotional intelligence, alongside engaging participants with the themes emerging from their experience of ill-health and the NHS.

> Arts activities can involve aesthetic engagement, involvement of the imagination, sensory activation, evocation of emotion and cognitive stimulation. Depending on its nature, an art activity may also involve social interaction, physical activity, engagement with themes of health. (Fancourt & Finn, 2019, p. 14)

Fancourt and Finn also claim that psychological, physiological, social and behavioural elements are all vital to using the arts in health care. In TBMA "psychological" refers to agency, coping and emotional regulation; "physiological" to less bodily distress from the symptom; "social" to reduced isolation, and social support; and "behavioural" to increased physical activity, healthier behaviours and self-management development.

The Intervention

Employing a facilitated group, and an embodied, enactive, expressive approach, is novel for MUS. It is not delivered one-to-one, nor as a group for a specific MUS condition as in CBT. Instead TBMA is delivered in a heterogenous group with people experiencing a variety of symptoms.

The TBMA specialist facilitator is crucial according to this study, although it is acknowledged the group support is also essential for efficacy, due to the population's extreme isolation. MUS sufferers feel they are the only one for whom their General Practitioner (GP) cannot find a diagnosis. They feel alone since friends/family have become bored of hearing about their symptoms, and often have less motivation to be active and go out, whereas a group promotes more engagement in life. They may feel helpless and hopeless (due to numerous tests and scans which come back normal). Participants are supported in challenging the notion of hopelessness and helplessness, giving a sense of agency. The arts are a perfect medium for combating social isolation, as well as developing agency and group cohesion. A group can generate new experiences and ideas for creativity, support and learning.

The intervention included 15 small groups delivered over 12 x 2 hourly sessions, over ten weeks. Individual consultations, before and after the group, took place with the group facilitator. Group numbers varied between four and ten.

Groupwork can be challenging for people, especially if already vulnerable, lacking confidence and highly anxious – often the case for people with MUS. Groups can be destructive, and access problematic, as research has shown (Smokowski, Rose & Bacallao, 2001). Consequently, strategies are employed prior to the group commencing to support people to engage and arrive at session one. For example, there is an individual intake meeting with the facilitator at the venue in the week before the first session. This explores people's fears, questions, provides ground rules/information and clarifies confidentiality. It engages the participant to find rapport/trust with the facilitator. Furthermore, participants only commit to attending six sessions initially, thereafter re-committing to the subsequent six, sustaining engagement more easily. Most participants attended regularly and completed the programme (97%). At the end there was an exit meeting, at which face-to-face semi-structured interviews or a participant experience form (PEF) were administered.

Methodology

The research question: "What are participants' perspectives on their experiences of TBMA?" The aim was to establish participants' experience of TBMA, and if any aspects of TBMA were helpful to developing the self-management of their symptoms.

This was a qualitative study evaluating post-programme perceptions from participants. Groups were delivered via different facilitators (N=3), in geographical areas and at different times. The qualitative findings reported here, derived from these deliveries, is consistent with the quantitative results previously published (Payne & Stott, 2010; Payne & Brooks, 2018) and provides rich data illustrating the process and understanding of the experience.

Data collection: There was a 65% (24/37) response rate. This research is a synthesis of qualitative data collected from face-to-face semi-structured interviews (which were recorded and transcribed) on participants' experiences of TBMA post intervention (N=18), combined with written qualitative data post-intervention from a PEF (N=24). The open-ended questions asked in the PEF were also based on the need to understand participants' experience of TBMA. The rich descriptive narratives describe participants' lived world experience of TBMA. The two sources of data collection (interviews plus PEF, N=42) provide for a method of cross-checking data to search for regularities and/or differences. The point of combining all perceptions was to create a larger number of perceptions.

Ethical approval: This was gained from the local NHS Research Ethics Committee for the data collection 2005–09 (number 05/Q0201/63). For subsequent data collection (2012–16) participants gave written consent to feedback/evaluations being used for research and could withdraw at any time without any reason. All participants agreed the data could be used for research purposes. Permission was gained from the NHS Clinical Commissioning Group to report on data anonymously in published articles. In all cases participants were assured of anonymity and confidentiality in the reporting without names or pseudonyms, i.e. only location and year of the group deliveries are referred to in participants' quotations.

Sample: Participants were drawn from patients suffering MUS in primary care in two clinical commissioning groups in the East of England. Recruitment for the groups was via GPs and self-referral confirmed by GPs. All participants presented in primary care with MUS for six months plus.

Gender: Of the 18 participants interviewed 15 were female and three were male. Of those participants who were invited to complete the PEF, 24 were returned out of which only 14 answered the question on gender. The gender mix, 8% male and 92% female, reflects the literature whereby more women than men somatise (Barsky, Peekna & Borus, 2001; Sowińska & Czachowski, 2018).

Ethnicity: Of those interviewed 18 reported being white, although not all British. Out of the 24 PEFs returned seven answered British white and 17 did not answer.

Age: Adults of all ages are likely to experience MUS. Of those interviewed, ages ranged from 21–81 years. Of those completing the PEF the biggest age category was 46–57 years. The youngest was 24 years and the eldest 63. One did not disclose date of birth.

Types of symptoms: There were 12 different symptoms for this data set of 12/18 patients:

☐ fatigue
☐ widespread chronic pain
☐ back pain
☐ left side pain
☐ lower back pain
☐ being cold
☐ movement restriction
☐ muscle hardening
☐ pain
☐ tiredness
☐ IBS
☐ anxiety

Employment status: There was data for only eight patients with a mixture of unemployed, retired and employed full or part time. For all deliveries most patients remained in the same employment. At the outset 1/8 (12%) of patients were retired; 0/8 (0%) were in full-time employment; 3/8 (38%) part time and 4/8 (50%) unemployed.

Educational background: Patients had a range of educational backgrounds, for example, none, A levels, degree level and post-graduate level. Socio-economic groups were not collected.

Inclusion/exclusion criteria:

Inclusion:

• 18 + years;
• MUS diagnosis for at least six months;
• frequent attender (four visits plus per annum);
• presentation for six months plus;

- co-morbid depression/anxiety;
- fluent English speaker.

Exclusion criteria:

- current relevant physical health problems;
- fewer than four GP consultations in previous year;
- trauma in previous six months;
- current relevant physical disability;
- complex bereavement in previous six months;
- learning disability;
- primary diagnosis of psychiatric condition in previous six months;
- current substance misuse;
- a diagnosed eating disorder.

Recruitment: There were two methods of recruitment. Health profession-als referring were aware of the nature of the research, the intervention and inclusion/exclusion criteria having attended a presentation and/or received a handout. They selected appropriate patients to whom to give a flyer and made a referral on their behalf. A second method was self-referral, for example, from notices in the community/GP surgery. Self-referrers completed a form reflecting inclusion/exclusion criteria and seeking permission to check suit-ability with GPs.

Procedures: For recruitment to groups, following referral on a first come first serve basis, patients received a leaflet about the learning group and then, if still interested, attended a half hour screening interview to establish suit-ability. Data for this aspect of the research was collected in the week the programme ended.

Analysis: The subsequent manual analysis of the PEF open-ended questions and the interview transcriptions resulted in several themes. Participants recounted examples of their experience of TBMA and ways in which they benefited. For the written responses the authors scrutinised the narratives identifying common themes and/or differences. Themes were derived from a step-by-step process of categorising quotations which related to specific content, tracking Braun and Clarke's (2006) approach to data analysis. This involved noting specific passages of text from the transcriptions and com-ments on the PEF linked by, or contrasting with, a common theme. This allowed the indexing of the text into categories to establish a framework of thematic ideas about the phenomena. By systematically interpreting and coding the textual data replicable and valid inferences were able to be made. Braun and Clarke's six steps were followed: familiarisation with data, gen-erating initial codes, searching for themes among codes, reviewing themes, defining and naming themes, and producing the final report. Five themes were identified and there follows a description of each theme in detail. These themes acted as proxy indicators for self-management.

This study employed a form of cross verification to check the credibility of the researchers' interpretation of the data, against the opinions of six different stakeholders engaged with the study (a referring GP, TBMA facilitators, the NHS commissioner, a non-involved researcher-practitioner with similar qualifications/experience, and one of the participants). In qualitative research, truthfulness can be assessed if the reader resonates with the outcomes as believable, consistent, applicable and useful to readers and other researchers. All stakeholders were invited to comment on the findings. One of the ways of enhancing validity is respondent validation: "a process whereby a researcher provides the people on whom he or she has conducted research with an account of his or her findings [in order to] seek corroboration or otherwise of the account" (Bryman, 2004, p. 274).

From the stakeholders' point of view there is some evidence for transferability to other settings. The reflexive translation into other contexts is where researchers/practitioners assess the extent to which findings in one context apply (or are transferable) to other contexts (Schofield, 1993). Hence, we also invited a research-practitioner to read the report, and assess the extent to which the intervention, and findings, could be applied to their context of MUS patients in primary care. Their assessment was that TBMA could be applied in such settings with resulting similar outcomes. Reliability (i.e. the consistency with which TBMA groups would produce the same findings) can be shown since the findings were derived from 15 groups of TBMA, with different facilitators, in different geographical regions, and yet were consistent.

Findings

Key for quotations: P=participant, P1=participant1, P2=participant2 in the same group/the initial letter of the venue used for the group and the number of the group in which the participant participated where relevant, i.e. 1 or 2/the year in which the group took place.

People enjoyed attending TBMA: 95% said they would recommend it to family and friends. The attrition rate was only 3%, and satisfaction rated good/very good on all aspects. It is noticeable participants mentioned elements which they took away from the experience of the intervention without commenting directly on the content of TBMA, which involved movement, dance and art-making practices; a common finding in similar interventions examining participants' views (Payne, 1986; Payne, 1996; Kaimal et al., 2019).

Categories were repeated and comments were plentiful showing saturation of patterns and repetitions. These were formed into five key principles presented here with one or two examples of participants' comments: 1) body with mind connections, 2) the importance of the facilitator, 3) positive benefits, 4) preparedness for change, and 5) self-acceptance/compassion. It is proposed that the interaction between these elements leads to an integration for self-management.

1. Body with mind connections

Movement and arts practices were designed to help people make connections between body and mind. People said they learned from witnessing others change their relationship with their symptoms/body. The term "BodyMind" derived from an analysis of participants' comments who, retrospectively, thought the workshop aim was to link the body with the mind – an aim which, they thought, had been met, for example: *"I learned to link my body with my mind"* (P, H3, 2008). This theme continued throughout the analysis, respondents commenting on how the embodied arts practices helped them find a voice and gain insight into their relationship with their body; listen to, and accept their energy levels; and use this monitoring to pace themselves, becoming more in touch with their body, *"Able to pace my day"* (P, HH, 2016) and *"Getting down to the root of the problem"* (P2, H, 2016). Links were made between feelings and symptom severity, and how mind tuned in with body giving more of an understanding of the relationship between body and mind. For example, they liked that *"the group was different in that they did unusual exercises like dancing, walking, breathing which helped me cope with my symptoms"* (P, H, 2013).

Participants reported listening to warning signals in the body which helped where symptoms can be addressed to learn how to *"live with the symptoms more easily"* (P, H3, 2008) as well as to *"learn how to cope with the symptoms"* (P, H3, 2008).

2. Importance of the facilitator

The data analysis led to the conclusion the facilitator was essential to the process engendering an inclusive and collaborative style, safety and support, and challenging participants to take risks. Participants commented the facilitators were very warm and understanding, knowledgeable, patient and helpful. For example: *"I learnt so much, and the facilitator is brilliant, she is patient, understanding and very knowledgeable"* (P, H4, 2016).

Some participants noted the facilitator created a safe environment, for example, for the changes required for self-management: *"I won't trust people easily but trusted the facilitator from day one"* (P, L1, 2015); *"Our leader was a great help in bringing about the group to gel from the start"* (P, H, 2013).

They thought the facilitator listened well, facilitated changes and gave freedom of choice/no pushing, helping people to learn how to open up. For example: *"[the facilitator] enforced or found boundaries, encouraging participants to listen to their inner voices*" (P1, H3, 2008). Additionally, they saw facilitators as being approachable, insightful and giving time to each person to be heard and understood. Some facilitators were also seen as nurturers, for example: "*She was nurturing or trying to caress them in a gentle way of exploring something that's quite painful for some people*" (P, H4, 2008); "*by providing safety (physically and emotionally) – nurturing the group*" (P, H3, 2008). It can be argued the non-judgemental, nurturing, kind attitudes demonstrated by facilitators helped people to open-up to self-compassion which is needed for self-management. The facilitator modelled the practices, joined in to lead dance/movement, and directed the mark-making for participants to engage with, and to link these to their symptom/s. Facilitators then guided discussion about symptoms and meanings derived from the embodied experience or artwork.

Facilitators were seen to help people learn how feelings are generated from themselves as opposed to from others – another aspect required for self-management. Participants explained the relationship with facilitators was profound, as "*a deep relationship*" enabling people to identify and express feelings giving tools to overcome symptoms: "*the fact we were given time to express our feelings was helpful*" (P, L2, 2015), as was "*positive encouragement and tools and space to overcome symptoms*" (P, H, 2013).

Facilitators helped participants to attribute new meaning to symptoms, i.e. turning bodily symptoms into meaningful information about current emotional states, typically saying: "*Realising my emotional situation is not helping my physical problems*" (P, H, 2015). Recognising these states, participants were guided by facilitators to inform themselves of their needs and ways to self-manage: "*I learned new ways of coping*" (P, H, 2013).

Facilitators convinced people to become interested in the meaning of their symptoms, and the part the symptom plays in their lives, accepting the symptom for what it is without judgement. The reward for learning is the continued capacity for growth, to go forward knowing they can be resilient in the face of adversity when it hits: "*[the facilitator] helped me find a way of moving forward*" (P, HH2, 2016).

Facilitator attributes include the ability to model staying in the present moment (Stern, 2004), for example: "*[the facilitator] helped me be more in the present*" (P, H4, 2008); "*[the facilitator] was excellent and always present*" (P2, L1, 2015); and "*[I] learned to be more present with me and symptoms*" (P, H3, 2008). This helped to promote connection with the body and the symptom to bring about self-management. Focusing on bodily sensation aids in the intention to be present, as well as focusing on the arts-making or movement process (as in adaptive authentic movement). Furthermore, creative experimentation with reference to the symptom in a safe environment – for example, creative movement with hands, reflective writing or mark-making – encourages an intention to stay with the present moment.

Facilitators engender and model non-judgemental and empathic attitudes, picked up by participants, to provide sufficient safety and support to open-up to playing, creativity, risk-taking and exploration. For example, "*I liked the fact it is free and non-judgemental*" (P, L1, 2015); another participant valued "*meeting others who had similar problems and not being judged*" (P, H, 2016).

3.   Positive benefits

From the data analysis it is concluded positive benefits from the arts practices in TBMA were feelings of a) belonging, b) support, c) safety and d) shared purpose, all of which are required to help develop the confidence to learn to self-manage. In a group each person brings the potential for rich experience whereby numerous perspectives are available. The experience in the group, and the group itself, was an important vehicle for change for almost all participants, for example: "*[it] worked like a catalyst*" (P, H2, 2008), or as a starting point offering an option: "*This group sort of showed me a road, and I could go down it, or not*" (P, H3, 2008) or "*[The] group supported me and helped me to accept the limits of my condition*" (P, L1, 2015).

The experience gave people a sense of belonging, "*Feeling less alone*" (P, H, 2016), as well as support and sharing: "*This course gave me the chance to unite, share experiences and support each other and gave a sense of belonging*" (P, L2, 2015). Discovering others with similar, or other, unexplained conditions helped feelings of belonging. Understanding they have had similar NHS experiences and seeing symptoms from new perspectives bonded people: "*being part of a group with people who are in a similar situation and learning to see your symptoms from a different angle*" (P, L1, 2015). Feelings of isolation reduced: "*I found getting other people's feedback and hearing their experiences helpful*" (P, L1, 2015). Participants made friends "*The group and our leader were all very friendly and helped each other, a good experience, I made a number of new friends, the group really gelled from the start*" (P, H, 2013). Participants mentioned they met group members post-course on a voluntary basis: "*I met people with a similar condition to myself and we are still meeting after it all ended*" (P, H, 2015). Seeing how others changed in their relationship to their body helped participants too: "*I have gained from the experience, particularly learning about my relationship with my body, and seeing it reflected in the others in the group*" (P, H, 2013).

4.   Preparedness for change

Participants appeared to be prepared to make changes, whereas previously they had resisted this. They reported on changes in their symptoms, lifestyle and mind-set (thinking) resulting from the experience of engaging with embodied experiments with the arts and creative movement. Such change could form the basis for self-management: "*I achieved a return to work and overcoming of fibromyalgia pains and symptoms in an on-going manner*" (P2, H, 2013).

Changes in thinking and habits developed, for example "*Changing thinking patterns and habits*" (P, H, 2016), as did changes in lifestyle: "*I was very set in a pattern, and it sort of acted as a catalyst to start my life changing, and it's changing more now, and quicker*" (P, H2, 2008). Mind-sets were also changed: "*a shift in outlook, a more positive approach*" (P, W, 2016); another participant "*facilitated a shift in how to manage [their] life*" (P, H2, 2008). All of these changes aid self-management. Hope for the future became important in the enbedment and maintenance of new habits, reduced worries and changed mind-sets, for sustaining self-management: "*I have been able to feel less worried and anxious about the future*" (P, S, 2016) and "*I feel more positive in my outlook and look forward to my future*" (P, L2, 2015). Mentioned frequently was the phrase "*I had enough help to go forward*" (P, L1, 2015). Other comments on hope for change included: "*I will find life more enjoyable since being involved with the facilitator and the group*" (P, L1, 2015).

Comments concerning change and choices included: "*I do take breaks and do whatever – silly things, but to give pleasure...jogging, listening to music or bubbling around somehow*" (P, H3, 2008); "*I question myself more before I commit myself to do so many things*" (P, H3, 2008).

Some participants referred to the change in reflections on the "self", with these statements concerning a deeper knowledge and understanding of self as a pre-requisite to change, for example: the programme "*[t]aught me a great deal about myself*" (P, L1, 2015); "*Questions I was asked made me look deeper into what was happening to me, making me think deep thoughts I had never realised needed looking into but have helped me very much*" (P, L2, 2015); and "*I [learned about] the inner self, to discover what you want and need (and to what extent)*" (P, H2, 2008).

Other comments were symptom related such as insight into the meaning or cause, developing coping strategies, and learning about their symptoms through the different art forms: "*[I learned] to find out more about the symptoms*" (P, H2, 2008). Flexibility and embracing the possibillity of change in their life emerged; some mentioned reduced anxiety/stress: "*improved stress management, therefore the symptom disappeared!*" (P, H4, 2008).

Participants thought the intervention had affected their lives both physically, such as feeling more energetic, relaxed and fitter, and in their overall wellbeing: "*My wellbeing has really improved generally*" (P, H1, 2008). Valuing one's self, indicating improved self-esteem, emerged – "*I now value myself and the quality of my life*" (P, H1, 2008) – and so did having more will power and self-reflection. For self-management there needs to be acknowledgement of physical change as well as self-reflection and motivation to sustain it. Ego strength provides the energy for self-agency and the ability to show it improved: "*I have direction now*" (P, L2, 2015); the programme "*enabled me to help myself*" (P1, H5, 2009). Another participant explained:

> [*The] activities taught has enabled me to control my anxiety and be more in tune with what my body needs. The many concepts and strategies taught have made me feel more empowered to tackle this illness and I am noticing a direct correlation between the level of anxiety and the severity of pain felt.* (P, W, 2016)

With reference to agency, it was not only about managing symptoms but also facilitating a shift in how to manage life and feeling more in control: "*more control of life, more structure/routine e.g. in family life*" (P, H3, 2008); "*It might give you your independence back from seeking medical advice all the time*" (P, H5, 2009). This would suggest that TBMA may save health service resources.

Other changes involving the management of feelings, characterised by comments such as "*I discovered that I get my symptoms through a lack of expressing how I feel*" (P, H4, 2008) and "*[I became able] to understand how worries can trigger symptoms*" (P, H5, 2009) show participants appear to have learned about repression, the influence of feelings on symptoms and the importance of expression as fostered by the embodied arts practices. Such learning can support strategies for self-management.

Participants found they had changed to be at the start of a journey: "*I feel I am only beginning this journey, as the changes I am putting in place will hopefully have an accumulative effect over time*" (P, H1, 2008). People said they were taking more time for fun things and breaks, or were making changes in diet to improve their stress levels. In terms of the sustainability of changes, a typical comment was: "*[the course] was life changing*" (P, H4, 2008).

Emphasising the change in positivity more readily appeared from a number of comments: "*friends have commented on how much I have improved with my positivity*" (P, S, 2016) and "*the course brought me to the point of 'I need to start living again' – it has helped me no end*" (P, W, 2016). The latter suggests life had been on hold due to MUS. Participants appeared to feel more empowered to tackle their illness, to start to do things for themselves such as meditation or painting, were more able to take on new things and found a way to move forward with self-care and less dependence on the NHS.

5. Self-acceptance/compassion

Self-acceptance and compassion derived from many comments. The symptom was transformed from being an "enemy" into an "ally" highlighting tolerance and acceptance – part of what is needed for self-management: "*I have become much more tolerant and understanding of my condition*" (P, S, 2016); "*It was a reminder to make time and space for myself, be more accepting and more relaxed*" (P, H, 2013); "*I have learned to accept it is OK to have limitations on what I can do*" (P, L2, 2015); "*Whilst I know the sessions won't cure my illness [...] I have learnt to accept it more, through different ways*" (P, H3, 2016); and "*[I] let go of my shame about my condition. [I am] in a much more accepting place which will help me achieve my goal of managing my energy better*" (P, L1, 2015) are good examples of this. Valuing the self is required for self-management: "*[I have] enhanced self-value, self-confidence*" (P, H1, 2008); one participant spoke of "*being kinder to self*" (P, W, 2016); and another "*learning to try and relax more and think about myself*" (P, H1, 2015).

Discussion

All these findings represent participants' take-home experience of the intervention in their terms. The content of sessions was based on arts and embodied practices as a means for exploring the symptom. Whilst participants have not specifically reported on these, they were the vehicle for experimentation and exploration to learn more about their symptoms, to provide a platform for self-management.

It is acknowledged MUS sufferers are hard-to-reach, perhaps because of the limited treatments acceptable to them; they are also hard to define and have varying levels of trust and confidence in the health service. TBMA appears to be a safe and non-threatening pathway to engaging this population.

Mobini (2015, p. 9) states, referring to patients' views, that "one of the major obstacles of delivering any psychological treatment to this clinical population is that often psychological treatment is considered as irrelevant and so referral to mental health services as unacceptable". TBMA appears to be seen by participants as relevant, as it is not framed as a psychological treatment but as a course of learning about symptoms and their management.

They may also be hard-to-reach due to the shame attached to being ill and/or sometimes absent from work with symptoms which are unexplained (inferring they are spurious, when they are real), for example, one participant said: "*I learned to let go of shame about my condition*" (P, L1, 2015). Such feelings of shame can be resolved if meaning can be attributed to the symptom, providing for a sense of control.

The themes above demonstrate several important ingredients and interrelating aspects for self-management. The following discussion for each of the five themes makes links to the literature.

1. Body with Mind Connections

The body with mind connection concept is a new and emerging area within the world-wide problem of MUS. Emotional processing involves both body and mind. For example, in patients with MUS/BDD, distancing practices in TBMA between emotion, symptom and self can cultivate more acceptance and greater understanding of the somatic experience. This in turn may afford the time and space to embrace other ideas and feelings which supplant the feelings of urgency to find a medical explanation. This could bring about a change in perspective and a different meaning of the symptom could become apparent. The new perspective towards the symptom can modulate feelings of urgency to find a cure/diagnosis. Once the feelings have been processed there can be a greater feeling of control, leading to new management strategies. The TBMA group can also support modulation of the urgency and provide opportunities for reflection on their own and others' experiences, with the group acting as a sounding board for ideas. With reference to this understanding, Town et al. (2019) conducted a small-scale study employing short-term dynamic psychotherapy exploring the contribution of emotional processing in the emergence, maintenance and experience of MUS.

Findings suggested internally observing the physical effects of emotional experiencing in MUS provides sensory evidence in the moment to enable patients to make mind-body connections. In TBMA the individual is nurtured towards engaging with their body symbolically, to view/experience it not only as a source of pain, discomfort and negative experiences, but also to acknowledge healthy, functioning aspects. Identifying sensations of symptoms, where they are in the body in a mindful way, with kind attention, leads to being able to control the distress. Sensations (interoception) are linked feelings and the imagination (via arts practices) and perception of the external environment in TBMA, raising body awareness to find meaning in the symptom.

Seeing others make connections between body and mind and making meaning of their symptoms can stimulate participants to make their own body with mind connections. Making these connections brings an appreciation of the ability to use bodily signals to self-regulate in a positive way, as opposed to previous, rather hostile, perspectives. TBMA promotes inhibition of old habits, reappraisal of pre-existing assumptions and possibilities to respond to stress in novel ways offering greater emotional self-regulation. Since emotions and movement are so closely related (Kirchhoff, 2018; Melzer, Shafir & Tsachor, 2019), non-verbal behaviour, as in expressive movement (Krantz & Pennebaker, 2007) and mark-making practices, can encourage reflections on a range of feelings (sadness, fear, anger, joy) which some people with MUS find difficult to identify and verbalise (alexithymia). This somatic, bottom-up intervention removes the focus on verbal language and memory, working with implicit elements available in the nonverbal. It appears the creative process, which involves play (Porges, 2015) within the group interactions, can lighten feelings of helplessness and hopelessness (Seligman & Groves, 1970).

Exploring the nature (or purpose) of the symptom, through experimenting with arts practices, creates distance between participant and symptom, allowing safety for meaningful aspects to emerge. Exploring sensorimotor experiences of symptoms, and employing grounding, mirroring and centring practices, can help reclaim emotional self-regulation and feelings of safety, leading to a greater sense of control.

2. *The Importance of the Facilitator*

Facilitators were perceived as catalysts, crucial for engendering hope for change. They were seen as knowledgeable specialists, role models, and a safe pair of hands, creating a safe, boundaried environment, helping people to open-up and feel comfortable, ensuring all were heard and understood. Participants felt safe enough to take the risks required to engage with the practices, and express feelings, since group cohesion (Forsyth, 2010) could be relied upon.

Facilitators honored symptoms, accepting them and the person unconditionally without judgement or questioning. Participants did not need to disclose their symptoms, but all were invited to bear their symptom in mind when engaging with practices. Symptoms were perceived as acting as agents for participants to listen to their own inner body-felt voices and address their problems. Facilitators valued participants' lived body experience, helping them to look at it afresh and focus on it as opposed to pushing it away as an enemy. Seeing, feeling and experiencing it "as is" rather than what they would like it to be, i.e. gone forever.

3. *Positive Benefits*

The benefits were feelings of a) belonging, b) support, c) safety and d) shared purpose. These were all present in TBMA groups and seemed important to the efficacy of TBMA according to participants. Cohesion is a general term for assessing the quality of the whole group, based on group integration and individual attraction to the group (MacKenzie, 1997; Dion, 2000). Participation increases in a cohesive group, and in return produces more interactions between members, leading to a more productive and effective group with better outcomes for its members and the group as a whole (Tschuschke & Dies 1994; Johnson & Johnson 2000; Marmarosh, Holtz & Schottenbauer, 2005; Marmarosh & Van Horn, 2010). Cohesion is regarded to be the most important process in a group (Yalom & Leszcz, 2005; Corey, 2004; Delucia-Waak & Bridboard, 2004; Brown & Lent, 2000). In TBMA cohesion refers to the quality of relationships that develop between group members and the facilitator (see 2 above) to promote a sense of "belonging", reducing isolation (Dirkzwager & Verhaak, 2007).

With reference to "support", participants commented on the significance of the individual members of the group, many opting to continue to meet voluntarily after the sessions and when the programme finished. Most participants commented that the interaction with group members improved wellbeing and gave a sense of support. For example, many arts practices took place individually (as in mark-making), in dyads (as in mirroring) or as a whole group when employing the Chace (1975) model of actively moving in synchrony to music together. After individually being engaged in an arts practice, participants would pair up to share and support one another. On other occasions participants would offer support to each other in the manner of witnessing, found in authentic movement (Whitehouse, 1999).

In TBMA groups "safety" is fundamental, and the programme is designed with that in mind (Payne & Brooks, 2019) since insecure attachment has been associated with MUS patients (Adshead & Guthrie, 2015). A positive perception of the group can indicate that members view the group as trustworthy and safe to explore and practise new skills within (Kivlighan & Tarrant, 2001). It is characterised by participants being active, engaged and seeing the group as beneficial. Orgodinsik and Piper (2003) indicated a correlation between short term group therapy, climate and outcomes, whether positive or negative depending on the level of conflict in the group and the phase of the group's development. However, in TBMA there is a trained facilitator to hold the group and curate its phases effectively, possibly speeding up the Tuckman's (1965) order, arriving at the stage of performing more swiftly.

Porges' (2003) Polyvagal Theory concludes that human social interaction combined with taking the mind-set into account in interventions turns off the sympathetic nervous system fight/flight/freeze response. The calming of the sympathetic system, combined with feeling listened to, enables people to feel "safe" enough to engage in the play required in TBMA arts practices, to do the work of self-reflection to achieve self-regulation and self-management (Porges, 2003). There appears to be an attitude of kind, loving acceptance in the group experience where all are equal and respected as individuals, adding to "safety" and experimentation. This contrasts with their views of previous experiences of unacceptance and disbelief surrounding symptoms. They may have been regarded as psychosomatic, confirming the symptoms are not genuine and, thus, their illness perceived as "illegitimate" (Kirmayer et al., 2004) and/or they should be able to fix it by themselves somehow (Kornelsen et al., 2016).

Participants perceived members as understanding and non-judgemental, as people shared experiences of symptoms, and the NHS as promoting a sense of "shared purpose". They had all joined the programme to learn more about their symptoms which already gave a shared purpose. It was never mentioned that the programme would cure symptoms but there was ambition that people could learn to self-manage them. Living with the unknown is extremely stressful; people can begin to imagine the worst, for example assuming they have the "big C". They also fear a mental health diagnosis since the assumption is that without a medical diagnosis all is imagined. One participant said at the first session "*If this group is about mental health, then*

I am leaving now!" Sharing experiences of symptoms normalises such fears and the MUS itself gives a shared sense of purpose too.

The experiences promoted change in symptom perception, coping styles, illness beliefs and personal dynamics – all necessary to achieve an increase in feelings of agency and control for self-management. Survival as a species is dependent upon the needs and experiences of others (Beckman & Syme, 1979). Hence there is dependence upon connecting. We have "evolved the capacity to feel social pains and pleasures, forever linking our well-being to our social connectedness. Infants embody this deep need to stay connected, but it is present through our entire lives" (Lieberman, 2013, p. 10). Furthermore, primates have developed an unparalleled ability to understand the actions and thoughts of those around them, enhancing their ability to stay connected and interact strategically. He goes on to say: "This capacity allows humans to create groups that can implement nearly any idea and to anticipate the needs and wants of those around us, keeping our groups moving smoothly" (Lieberman, 2013, p. 10). Although the self may appear to be a mechanism for distinguishing us from others, and perhaps accentuating our selfishness, the self operates as a powerful force for social cohesiveness. "Whereas connection is about our desire to be social, harmonising refers to the neural adaptations that allow group beliefs and values to influence our own" (Lieberman, 2013, p. 11). The embodied, expressive movement experiences in TBMA engender the social connectedness/bonds to facilitate the shared purpose of learning more about symptoms.

TBMA groups share a purpose, practices, values and beliefs and these can influence each member of the group positively. We propose the outcome of self-agency, required for self-management, is derived from the social construction developed from confidence gained from the group's shared purpose, support, sense of belonging and safety.

Physiologically, although the intervention did not suggest it would cure or reduce symptom distress, many participants commented on how their symptoms had reduced or disappeared. Pain, particularly, was reported to have decreased.

4.   *Preparedness for Change*

Cohesion in the group leads to more risk taking in giving feedback and establishing interpersonal relationships (Yalom & Leszcz, 2005). Risk taking leads to change in a group setting (Greer, 2012). TBMA encourages risk taking and therefore opportunities for change in a safe, interactive environment. For example, self-disclosure, feedback and the contributions of the facilitator and group members all reflect risk taking and increase cohesion in the group (Burlingame, McLendon & Alonso, 2011). Research suggests cohesion plays a role in the outcomes of groups (Brown & Lent, 2000). In TBMA there was a shift, according to participants, to becoming more positive for hope for change for the better and a belief that change was possible (i.e. to self-manage symptoms). Kivlighan et al. (2016) found a significant relationship between an individual member's post treatment hope and the aggregated sense of hope of other group members. Participants reported new habits, feelings, routines, lifestyle and mind-set (Wood & Runger, 2016), all of which are required for self-management. Self-understanding and making meaning appeared to be pre-requisites when making changes.

Participants described the group as life-changing, describing reduced anxiety about the future, improved stress management and regaining interest in past pursuits. Participants reported improved physical and mental wellbeing; enhancing self-esteem, willpower and self-regulation; pacing themselves better; and cultivating healthier routines. Recognising feelings, as well as understanding their relationship with symptoms and triggers for their symptoms and emotions, was important in the group. Links were made between emotions, thoughts, feelings and the sensation of symptoms.

Change was described as the beginning of a journey, and the belief expressed that the improvement can accumulate over time, with on-going conscious and/or unconscious impact. Some people felt empowered to tackle their illness, noticing a relationship between anxiety and pain. La Cour and Petersen (2015) found an association between anxiety and pain relief. All this points to the capacity to learn hope for the future and take some control, as opposed to their previous state of learned helplessness (Seligman & Groves, 1970).

Role play (Corsini, 2017) is both part of the group experience and a practice in TBMA. For example, asking participants to share in pairs how their symptom may move or the posture it might take up. This often leads to greater insight into the meaning of symptoms. The languaging of the feeling state in such a posture, for example, might contribute to a greater meaning-making of its nature and role in life. Feedback received from their partner could add further to this meaning. For example, a participant saw the image of a lion emerge from sensing her symptom through non-directed, expressive bodily movement, which she interpreted as anger. During the verbal dyad process her partner also saw features of this animal. The dialogue that followed between them helped this participant to consider how to moderate her anger which she realised tended to trigger her symptoms. The participant dialogued with their symptoms to explore and better understand, re-frame or gain an explanation of meaning, origins, triggers and maintenance of them day-to-day.

Confidence gained in the group enabled the reduction of shame, improved wellbeing, self-esteem and the capacity to believe things could change for the better, promoting the development of a mind-set to embrace change and self-management skills.

5. Self-Acceptance/Self-Compassion

Participants began to accept their symptoms as a part of themselves, rather than fearing them and wanting to be free of them, which brought some emotional release. They seemed to realise their symptom will not harm them or be a threat which indicates a change from seeing their symptom as a foe to becoming a friend reducing the attempts to be symptom-free.

Finding the capability for self-compassion is accompanied by a sense of prioritising the body's needs and bringing a sense of ease. Through the accepting ethos offered by TBMA participants are afforded the opportunity to learn the value of self and others. Self-acceptance/compassion was concerned with understanding other participants' conditions and having a tolerance of them, with kindness. This then became self-compassion; for example, the notion of accepting the symptom, non-judgementally, appeared in the data often. The pathway appears to have travelled from accepting the symptom to accepting the self, to self-compassion allowing the participant to relax into their body/bodily symptoms in a more accepting way. This contributes to an ending of the fight between person and symptom or mind and body respectively. The search for a cure/explanation medically or psychologically is no longer such an imperative. Arriving at this place of acceptance and cultivating self-compassion was found to be the strongest mechanism of change in several other studies (van Ravesteijn et al., 2014; Pourova et al., 2020). Lind et al. (2014) found relevant themes, specifically the need for recognition of symptoms (believed by others, which helps towards self-acceptance.

Rohricht et al. (2019) used dance movement psychotherapy in an RCT. Results from self-report standardised questionnaires demonstrated a significant reduction in symptom severity and gain in quality of life, continuing at six-months post-intervention interviews. They suggest the process of change involves an element of self-acceptance and better coping strategies.

Van Ravesteijn et al. (2014) examined the effectiveness of mindfulness based cognitive therapy (MBCT) using grounded theory to construct a process of change. Twelve semi-structured interviews were analysed demonstrating the process of change to be circular and iterative rather than linear. Acceptance was viewed as an essential step in the process of moving back and forth between stages and at different paces, with the change arising from being more self-compassionate. In this study the process of change was determined by: a) attention regulation (attending to the present moment), b) increased body awareness (noticing arising bodily sensations), c) emotion regulation (recognising the inter-connectedness of emotions and thoughts) and d) change in how they view the self. Patients are usually fearful and stressed about their symptoms and want to get rid of them.

This causes the constant searching for answers and cures which maintains an emotional state of anxiety. Hence, "no news" on the medical diagnosis is not the "good news" that one might expect. On the other hand, becoming less fearful and more accepting of their symptoms (i.e. that they will not harm themselves) relieves them from a state of anxiety and/or depression so prevents the downward spiral and ignites an upward one. The programme for TBMA enables them to reach a place of self-compassion and make adaptations to life, easing living with their symptoms/living well despite the symptoms. Being more connected to their body appeared to allow a greater capacity to notice energy limits and when to rest/relax. Sharing experiences in the group helped participants gain a perspective of their own situation. Journaling provided enforced time to reflect on experiences each session. Participants learned, for example, it was acceptable to have limitations allowing them to accept what their body tells them it needs. Comments on outcomes included enhanced self-value and self-confidence changing the mind-set to one of self-compassion.

Of the mechanisms of change in Pourova et al. (2020), over 67 studies, those receiving most support were 1) increasing symptom acceptance, 2) developing coping strategies and 3) positive treatment expectations. They included studies focusing on single diagnoses, such as CFS. These three mechanisms resonate with elements of TBMA such as acceptance of self and of symptoms and the notion of action plans which embody coping strategies as an outcome from TBMA for self-care going forward. The session attendance figures for the groups could be seen as anticipation the intervention would be beneficial.

The honesty encouraged by the facilitator in the group nurtures people to accept the idea they have a condition which, although may not be curable, is something they can learn to manage. It should be noted in some cases symptoms did disappear. Finally, acceptance (of their condition) in the supportive group and self-acceptance/compassion appears to be key to starting to self-manage (Gregg et al., 2007), as opposed to seeking a cure, from the health service. The group promoted greater understanding of the condition and the acceptance of the lack of a cure; these can be helped with an explanatory model which can kick-start change, and obviate the need for more tests and scans. Learning through the group to become kinder to the self reflects an important attitude to developing self-management. Acceptance of self, own needs and symptoms are a pre-requisite for self-managing symptoms changing the mind-set from "I am not OK" to "I am OK", (Harris, 1970) despite symptoms and limitations.

The changes made to TBMA over the years were only structural, for example, omitting assessments halfway through the programme, or front-loading sessions to twice weekly for the first two weeks to facilitate group cohesion and engagement. The reason for a few changes is that TBMA is not a prescriptive model, setting out tasks per session as with other structured programmes. Trained facilitators will modify TBMA interventions to the group needs but within a known framework with topics to be covered, the tailoring of which is down to the professional judgement of the facilitator, i.e. TBMA responds to the group rather than the group having to adhere to it. Having said that, there is a manual, and facilitator training is standardised in that it is delivered by the same trainers, and with the same content, adjusted as would be expected, depending on trainees' needs. There is an assessment process for certification.

After the first two weeks the groups became closed to new participants and remained constant. Group size appears to have been relatively unimportant, probably because the facilitator was responsive to the needs of each group, irrespective of size. The smaller groups did miss those absent at times, there was some depletion of the richness due to this.

We employed dance movement psychotherapists rather than other professional psychotherapists, since they would have knowledge, skills and experience of body-centred exercises and understand the body with mind interdependency. Although TBMA does employ elements from all the arts, specialists in other therapies may have different skills, for example, music, talking or art therapists.

Potential limitations were the small numbers of participants, the limited amount interviewed (N=20), all groups conducted in one south of England middle-class area, and the need for more trained facilitators and groups. Funding was also limited.

Recommendations for further research would include addressing the above limitations in a larger qualitative study. Additionally, a quantitative or mixed methodology study, further to Payne and Brooks (2017), would ideally include a control cohort, and be conducted in more than one region of England.

Summary

This was a qualitative study to discover participants' perceptions of the experience of TBMA.

We were not evaluating in the quantitative paradigm to discover whether outcomes were as a result of the group or arts experience, therefore there no control group was required. The research was based on an analysis of qualitative data and notes five consistent themes we call key principles: body with mind connections; the importance of the facilitator; positive benefits; preparedness change; and acceptance/compassion. These all appear to have kickstarted the self-management process for participants.

These five key principles in TBMA demonstrate several important ingredients and inter-relating aspects for the self-management of MUS. It is possible to distinguish the success of TBMA from the influence of the facilitator because there were several different facilitators, delivering in different regions, at different times, with different groups of people and yet all groups demonstrated similar outcomes. The perceptions arose from open-ended questions about the programme which did not focus on the arts practices per se, independent of the group and the group experience. However, because the arts practices were integral to the group experience it is reasonable to infer the perceptions reported connected to these practices. It seems likely, therefore, due to the holistic, integrative nature of TBMA, that all these elements may be involved.

We have outlined a model highlighting the interaction between the five key principles in TBMA. It shows how TBMA, with its emphasis on the arts, bodily sensations, creativity and expressive, movement-based embodied contemplative practices, in a facilitated group setting can help to re-establish sensorimotor integration. Furthermore, TBMA can foster non-judgmental, compassionate and accepting attitudes leading towards a reconnection with bodily sensations, improved self and body confidence, functionality and quality of life. These findings expand the scope of reflection regarding the relationship between the arts, body awareness and MUS, including interoceptive and emotional aspects of the MUS BodyMind relationship. It takes further the idea of self-management from its employment with identified diseases, to its adoption as a strategy for management and treatment of MUS, which currently have poor outcomes. TBMA may be transferable to other long-term conditions in health education settings.

The potential benefits of TBMA to support patients with MUS to learn to self-manage could mean that it replaces current treatments (which are unacceptable to patients) and integrates the body and mind in one holistic biopsychosocial model. Furthermore, it could reduce the high costs for MUS conditions, freeing up GP time, increasing capacity and resources. The programme is unique in its potential reach, significance and impact since MUS is ubiquitous.

This study is relevant to health care as well as to dance movement psychotherapy. Benefits from participation in TBMA were feelings of belonging, support, safety and shared purpose, all important for people in distress. Facilitated group experience is a vehicle for change and the use of TBMA makes it even stronger.

Funding

The study (2005–09) was funded by the East of England Development Agency and the University of Hertfordshire and data collected 2012–16 was funded by the Department of Health QIPP programme and East and North Herts and Herts Valleys Clinical Commissioning Groups.

Acknowledgements

The authors are grateful to the participants, facilitators and funders without whom this research would not have been conducted. Special thanks go to the people who assessed and validated the findings (testimonies available on request) on the following criteria: (1) believability, (2) consistency, (3) applicability and transferability and (4) credibility. Facilitators, a practitioner-researcher, a commissioner, a GP and a patient suffering MUS who attended the programme all read and assessed the findings and have given their permission to be acknowledged here: Doe Warnes, Louis Sandford, Silvana Reynolds, Mira Schauble, Simon Chatfield and Lynn Boyden.

References

Adler, J. (2002). *Offering from the Conscious Body: The Discipline of Authentic Movement*. Inner Traditions Bear and Co.

Adshead, G., and Guthrie, E. (2015). The role of attachment in medically unexplained symptoms and long-term illness. *British Journal of Psychological Advances*, 21(3), 167–174. doi: 10.3389/fpsyg.2019.01818

APPG. (2017). Creative Health: The Arts for Health and Wellbeing. London: All-Party Parliamentary Group on Arts, Health and Wellbeing. http://www.artshealtha ndwellbeing.org.uk/appg-inquiry/ Accessed 15 January 2020.

Barsky, A. J., Peekna, H. M., and Borus, J. F. (2001). Somatic symptom reporting in women and men. *Gen. Intern. Med.* Apr; 16(4): 266–275. doi: 10.1046/j.1525-1497.2001.00229.x

Beckman, L. F., and Syme, S. L. (1979). Social networks, host resistance and mortality: A new year follow-up study of Alameda County residents. *American Journal of Epidemiology*, 109, 186–204. doi: 10.1093/oxfordjournals.aje.a112674

Beebe, B., and Lachmann, F. (1998). Co-constructing inner and relational processes: Self and mutual regulation in infant research and adult treatment. *Psychoanal. Psychol.*, 15, 1–37.

Bermingham, S. L., Cohen, A., Hague, J., and Parsonage, M. (2010). The cost of somatization among the working-age population in England for the year 2008–2009. *Mental Health Family Medicine*, 7(2), 71–84.

Bjørnnes, A. K., Parry, M., and Leegaard, M. (2018). Self-management of cardiac pain in women: A meta-summary of the qualitative literature. *Qualitative Health Research*, 28(11), 1769–1787. https://doi.org/10.1177/1049732318780683

Braun, V., and Clarke, V. (2006). Using thematic analysis in psychology. *Qualitative Research in Psychology*, 3(2), 77–101.

Brown, S. D., and Lent, R. W. (Eds) (2000). *Handbook of Counselling Psychology*, 3rd edn. Wiley.

Bryman, A. (2004). *Social Research Methods*, 2nd edn. Oxford University Press.

Burton, C., McGorm, K., … and Sharpe, M. (2012) Healthcare costs incurred by patients repeatedly referred to secondary medical care with medically unexplained symptoms: A cost of illness study. *Psychosomatic Research*, 72(3), 242–247. doi:10.1016/j.jpsychores.2011.12.009

Chace, M. (1975). Untitled article on professional history. In H. Chaiklin (Ed.), *Marian Chace: Her Papers*. American Dance Therapy Association.

Challis, D., Hughes, J., Berzins, K., Reilly, S., Abell, J., and Stewart, K. (2010). *Self-care and case management in long-term conditions: The effective management of critical interfaces*. Social Services Research Unit, SDO Project (08/1715/201) http://www.pssru.ac.uk/pdf/MCpdfs/SCCMfr.pdf

Chew-Graham, C. A., Heyland, S., ... and Sumathipala, A. (2017), Medically unexplained symptoms: continuing challenges for primary care. *Br. J. Gen. Pract.* Mar; 67(656), 106–107. doi: 10.3399/bjgp17X689473. Erratum in: *Br. J. Gen. Pract.* 2019 Jul; 69(684), 333. doi: 10.3399/bjgp19X704285.

Corey, G. (2004). *Theory and Practice of Group Counselling*, 6th edn. Thomson/Brooks/Cole Publishing.

Corsini, R. (2017). *Role Playing in Psychotherapy*. Aldine.Delucia-Waack., D. A. Gerrity., C. R. Kalodner., and M. T. Riva (Eds), *Handbook of Group Counselling and Psychotherapy* (pp. 120–135). Sage.

Delucia-Waack, J. L., and Bridbord, K. H. (2004). Measures of group process, dynamics, climate, leadership behaviours, and therapeutic factors: A review. In J. L.

Department of Health. (2008). Improving Access to Psychological Therapies. MedicallyUnexplained Symptoms Positive Practice Guide, www.iapt.nhs.uk

Dion, K. L. (2000). Group cohesion: From "field of forces" to multidimensional construct. *Group Dynamics: Theory, Research, and Practice*, 4(1), 7–26. http://dx.doi.org/10.1037/1089-2699.4.1.7

Dirkzwager, A. J., Verhaak, O. F. (2007). Patients with persistent medically unexplained symptoms in general practice: characteristics and quality of care. *BMC Family Practice*, May 31; 8: 33. https://doi.org/10.1186/1471-2296-8-33

Eberhard-Kaechele, M. (2019). A developmental taxonomy of interaction modalities in dance movement therapy. In: H. Payne, S. Koch, S., J. Tantia with T. Fuchs (Eds.,). *The Routledge International Handbook of Embodied Perspectives in Psychotherapy* (pp. 81–95). Routledge.

Fancourt, D. and Finn, S. (2019). *What Is the Evidence on the Role of the Arts in Improving Health and Well-Being? A Scoping Review*. Health Evidence Network (HEN) synthesis report. Copenhagen: WHO Regional Office for Europe.

Fink, P., and Schroder, A. (2010). One single diagnosis, bodily distress syndrome, succeeded to capture 10 diagnostic categories of functional somatic syndromes and somatoform disorders. *Psychosomatic Research*, 68, 415–426. doi:10.1016/j.jpsychores.2010.02.004

Fogel, A. (1993). *Developing Through Relationships*. University of Chicago Press.

Fonagy, P., Gergely, G., Jurist, E. L., and Target, M. (2002). *Affect Regulation, Mentalization, and the Development of the Self*. Other Press.

Forsyth, D. R. (2010). *Group Dynamics*, 5th edn (pp. 118–122). Wadsworth Cengage Learning.

Gallagher, S. (2019). Precis: Enactivist Interventions. *Philosophical Studies*, 176, 803–806. https://doi.org/10.1007/s11098-018-01230-8

Greer, L. L. (2012). Group cohesion: Then and now. *Small Group Research*, 43(6), 655–661. https://doi.org/10.1177/1046496412461532

Gregg, J., Callaghan, G. M., Hayes, S. C., and Glenn-Lawson, J. L. (2007). Improving diabetes self-management through acceptance, mindfulness, and values: A randomized controlled trial. *Journal of Consulting and Clinical Psychology*, 75, 2, 336–343. doi:10.1037/0022-006X.75.2.336.

Haller, H., Cramer, H., Lauche, R. and Dobos, G. (2015). Somatoform disorders and medically unexplained symptoms in primary care: A systematic review and meta-analysis of prevalence. *Dtsch Arztebl Int.* 112(16): 279–287. doi:10.3238/arztebl.2015.0279

Harris, T. (1970). *I'm OK – You're OK*. Pan publications.

Hart, Y., Noy, L., Feniger-Schaal, R., Mayo, A. E., and Alon, U. (2014). Individuality and togetherness in joint improvised motion. *PloS ONE*, 9(2), e87213. https://doi.org/10.1371/journal.pone.0087213

Henningsen, P., Zipfel, S., and Herzog, W. (2007). Management of functional somatic syndromes. *Lancet*, 369(9565), 946–955. doi:10.1016/S0140-6736(07)60159-7

Johnson, D. W. and Johnson F. P. (2000). *Joining Together: Group Theory and Group Skills*, 7th edn. Allyn and Bacon.

Kaimal, G., Jones, J. P., Dieterich-Hartwell. R., Acharya, B., and Wang, X. (2019). Evaluation of long- and short-term art therapy interventions in an integrative care setting for military service members with post-traumatic stress and traumatic brain injury. *The Arts in Psychotherapy*, 62, 28–36.

Kirchhoff, M. (2018). The body in action: predictive processing and the embodiment thesis In A. Newen, L. De Bruin and S. Gallagher (Eds), *Oxford Handbook of 4E Cognition* (Chapter 12). Oxford University Press.

Kirmayer, L. J., Groleau, D., Looper, K.J., and Dao M. D. (2004). Explaining medically unexplained symptoms. *Canadian Journal of Psychiatry*, 49(10), 663–72. doi: 10.1177/070674370404901003.

Kivlighan, D. M., Paquin, J. D., Hsu, Y. K. K., and Wang, L. (2016). The mutual influence of therapy group members' hope and depressive symptoms. *Small Group Research*, 47(1), 58–76. doi.org/10.1177/1046496415605638

Kivlighan, D. M., Jr., and Tarrant, J. M. (2001). Does group climate mediate the group leadership–group member outcome relationship? A test of Yalom's hypotheses about leadership priorities. *Group Dynamics: Theory, Research, and Practice*, 5(3), 220–234. http://dx.doi.org/10.1037/1089-2699.5.3.220

Kornelsen, J., Atkins, C., Brownell, K., and Woollard, R. (2016). The meaning of patient experiences of medically unexplained physical symptoms. *Qualitative Health Research*, 26(3), 367–376. doi: 10.1177/1049732314566326.

Krantz, A. M., and Pennebaker, J. W. (2007). Expressive dance, writing, trauma and health: when words have a body. In I. A. Serlin, J. Sonke-Henderson, R. Brandman, and J. Graham-Pole (Eds.), *Praeger Perspectives. Whole Person Healthcare Vol. 3. The Arts Health* (p. 201–229). Praeger Publishers.

la Cour, P., and Petersen, M. (2015). Effects of mindfulness meditation on chronic pain: a randomized controlled trial. *Pain Medicine*, 16(4), 641–652.

Lieberman, M. D. (2013). *Social. Why Our Brains Are Wired to Connect*. Oxford University Press.

Lind, A. B., Delmar, C., and Nielsen, K. (2014). Searching for existential security: a prospective qualitative study on the influence of mindfulness therapy on experienced stress and coping strategies among patients with somatoform disorders. *J. Psychosom. Res*. Dec; 77(6), 516–521. doi: 10.1016/j.jpsychores.2014.07.015

MacKenzie, K. R. (1997). Clinical application of group development ideas. *Group Dynamics: Theory, Research, and Practice*, 1(4), 275–287. https://doi.org/10.1037/1089-2699.1.4.275

Marmarosh, C., Holtz, A., and Schottenbauer, M. (2005). Group cohesiveness, group-derived collective self-esteem, group-derived hope, and the well-being of group therapy members. *Group Dynamics: Theory, Research, and Practice*, 9, 32–44. doi:10.1037/1089-2699.9.1.32

Marmarosh, C. L., and Van Horn, S. M. (2010). Cohesion in counselling and psychotherapy groups. In R. K. Conyne (Ed.), *The Oxford Handbook of Group Counselling* (pp. 137–163) Oxford University Press.

Melzer, A., Shafir, T. and Palnick Tsachor, R. (2019). How do we recognize emotion from movement? Specific motor components contribute to the recognition of each emotion. *Front. Psychol.*, 10:1389. https://doi.org/10.3389/fpsyg.2019.01389

Miller, W. L. and Crabtree, B. F. (2005). Clinical research. In: N. Denzin and Y. Lincoln (Eds) *Handbook of Qualitative Research*, 3rd edn. Sage Publications.

Mobini, S. (2015). Psychology of medically unexplained symptoms: A practical review, *Cogent Psychology*, 2, 1, doi: 10.1080/23311908.2015.1033876

Nimnuan, T., Hotopf, M., and Wessely, S. (2001). Medically unexplained symptoms: An epidemiological study in seven specialties. *Psychosomatic Research*, 51(1): 361–367. doi: 10.1016/s0022-3999(01)00223-9.

Orgodinsik, J., and Piper, W. (2003). The effect of group climate on outcome in two forms of short-term group therapy. *Group Dynamics: Theory, Research and Practice*, 7, 64–76. doi:10.1037/1089-2699.7.1.64

Pallaro, P. (Ed.) (2007). *Authentic Movement: Moving the Body, Moving the Self, Being Moved. A Collection of Essays*. Volume 2. Jessica Kingsley.

Payne, H. (1986). Dance Movement Therapy with Adolescents Labelled Delinquent. University of Manchester, thesis submission in partial fulfilment of M. Phil.

Payne, H. (1996). A Personal Development Group in Therapy Training in Higher Education. University of London, thesis submitted in partial fulfilment of a Ph.D.

Payne, H. (2006). The body as container and expresser: Authentic Movement groups in the development of wellbeing in our bodymindspirit. In: J. Corrigall, H. Payne and H. Wilkinson (Eds,) *About a Body: Working with the Embodied Mind in Psychotherapy* (pp. 162–181). Routledge.

Payne, H. (2009a). Medically unexplained conditions and the BodyMind approach. *Counselling in Primary Care Review*, 10, 1, 6–8.

Payne, H. (2009b). Pilot study to evaluate Dance Movement Psychotherapy (the BodyMind Approach) with patients with medically unexplained symptoms: participant and facilitator perceptions and a summary discussion. *Int. J. Body, Movement and Dance in Psychotherapy*. 5, 2, 95–106. https://doi.org/10.1080/1743297090 2918008

Payne, H., and Brooks, S. D. M. (2017). Moving on: The BodyMind Approach for medically unexplained symptoms. *Journal of Public Mental Health*, 16(2), 1–9. doi: 10.1108/JPMH-10-2016-0052

Payne, H. and Brooks, S. (2019) Medically unexplained symptoms and attachment theory: The BodyMind Approach®, *Frontiers in Psychology, Section Psychology for Clinical Settings*, 10, 1818. https://doi.org/10.3389/fpsyg.2019.01818

Payne, H., Jarvis, J. and Roberts, A. (2020) The BodyMind Approach as transformative learning to promote self-management for patients with medically unexplained symptoms.*Transformative Education*, 18(2) 114–137. https://doi.org/10.1177/1541344619883892

Payne, H., and Stott, D. (2010). Change in the moving bodymind: Quantitative results from a pilot study on the BodyMind Approach (TBMA) as groupwork for patients with medically unexplained symptoms (MUS). *Counselling and Psychotherapy Research*, 10, 4, 295–307. https://doi.org/10.1080/14733140903551645

Porges, S. (2003). Social engagement and attachment: a phylogenetic perspective. *Annals of New York Academy of Sciences*, 1008. 31–47. doi: 10.1196/annals.1301.004.

Porges, S. (2015). Play as a neural exercise: insights from the Polyvagal Theory. In D. Pearce-McCall (Ed.,), *The Power of Play for Mind Brain Health* (pp. 3–7).

Pourová, M., Klocek, A., Řiháček, T., and Čevelíček, M. (2020). Therapeutic change mechanisms in adults with medically unexplained physical symptoms: a systematic review. *Psychosomatic Research*, 134: 110124. doi:10.1016/j.jpsychores.2020.110124

Purdy, S. (2010). *Avoiding Hospital Admissions. What Does the Research Evidence Say?* The Kings Fund, December, 2010. http://www.kingsfund.org.uk/publications/avoiding_hospital.html

Rabinowitch T. C., Meltzoff A. N. (2017). Synchronized movement experience enhances peer cooperation in preschool children. *Exp. Child Psychol.* 160 2132.10.1016/j.jecp.2017.03.001.

Rennung, M., and Göritz, A. S. (2016). Prosocial consequences of interpersonal synchrony: A meta-analysis. *Zeitschrift für Psychologie*, 224(3), 168–189. http://dx.doi.org/10.1027/2151-2604/a000252

Rohricht, F., Sattel, H., Kuhn, C., and Lahmann, C. (2019). Group body psychotherapy for the treatment of somatoform disorder – a partly randomised-controlled feasibility pilot study. *BMC Psychiatry*, 19: 120. https://doi.org/10.1186/s12888-019-2095-6

Schofield, J. W. (1993) Increasing the generalizability of qualitative research. In M. Hammersley (Ed.,), *Educational Research: Current Issues*, London: Paul Chapman.

Schore, A. N. (2003). *Affect Regulation and the Repair of the Self*. Norton.

Schore, A., and Schore, J. R. (2006). *Reader's Guide to Affect Regulation and Neurobiology: A Desktop Reference to the Terms and Concepts in this Burgeoning Field*. Norton.

Seligman, M. E. P., and Groves, D. (1970). Non-transient learned helplessness. *Psychonomic Science*, 19, 191–192. https://doi.org/10.3758/BF03335546

Shim, R. M., Johnson, B … and Bradt, J. (2017). A model of dance/movement therapy for resilience-building in people living with chronic pain. *European Journal of Integrative Medicine*, 9, 27–40, https://doi.org/10.1016/j.eujim.2017.01.011.

Siegal, D. J. (2012). *Pocket Guide to Interpersonal Neurobiology: An Integrative Handbook of the Mind*. W. W. Norton Co.

Smokowski, P. R., Rose, S. D., and Bacallao, M. L. (2001). Damaging experiences in therapeutic groups: how vulnerable consumers become group casualties. *Small Group Research*, 32(2), 223–251. doi.org/10.1177/1

Sowińska, A., and Czachowski, S. (2018). Patients' experiences of living with medically unexplained symptoms (MUS): a qualitative study. *BMC Fam. Pract.*, 19, 23. https://doi.org/10.1186/s12875-018-0709-6

Steinbrecher N., Koerber S., Frieser D., and Hiller W. (2011). The prevalence of medically unexplained symptoms in primary care. *Psychosomatics*, May–Jun; 52(3), 263–271. doi: 10.1016/j.psym.2011.01.007.

Stern, D. (2004). *The Present Moment in Psychotherapy and Everyday Life*. W.W. Norton Co.

Swartz, A. I. (2012). Embodied learning and patents education from nurses' self-awareness to patient self-caring. *New Directions for Adult and Continuing Education*, 1, 134, 15–24.

Tarr, B., Launay, J., and Dunbar, R. I. (2016). Silent disco: dancing in synchrony leads to elevated pain thresholds and social closeness. *Evolution and Human Behavior*, 37(5), 343–349. doi: 10.1016/j.evolhumbehav.2016.02.004

Town, J. M., Lomax, V., Abbass, A. A., & Hardy, G. (2019). The role of emotion in psychotherapeutic change for medically unexplained symptoms. *Psychotherapy Research*, 29(1), 86–98. https://doi.org/10.1080/10503307.2017.1300353 first published online (2017).

Tschuschke, V., and Dies, R. R. (1994). Intensive analysis of therapeutic factors and outcome in long-term inpatient groups. *Int. J. Group Psychotherapy*, Apr; 44(2), 185–208. doi: 10.1080/00207284.1994.11490742.

Tuckman, B. W. (1965). Developmental sequence in small groups. *Psychological Bulletin*, 63, 384–399. https://doi.org/10.1037/h0022100

van Ravesteijn, H. J., Yvonne, B., … and Speckens, C. (2014) Mindfulness-based cognitive therapy (MBCT) for patients with medically unexplained symptoms: Process of change, *Psychosomatic Research*, 77, 1, 27–33, https://doi.org/10.1016/j.jpsychores.2014.04.010

Vicaria, I. M., and Dickens, L. (2016). Meta-analyses of the intra- and interpersonal outcomes of interpersonal coordination. *Nonverbal Behavior*, 40, 335–361. https://doi.org/10.1007/s10919-016-0238-8

Whitehouse, M. (1999). Creative expression in physical movement is language without words. In: P. Pallaro, (Ed.,), *Authentic Movement: Essays by Mary Starks Whitehouse, Janet Adler and Joan Chodorow*. Jessica Kingsley Publications.

Wood, W., and Runger, D. (2016). Psychology of habit. *Annual Review of Psychology*, 67, 289–314. https://doi.org/10.1146/annurev-psych-122414-033417

Yalom, I. D., and Leszcz, M. (2005). *The Theory & Practice of Group Psychotherapy*, 5th edn. Basic Books.

Chapter 7

Addressing Insecure Attachment Patterns

(A version of this chapter was first published in *Frontiers in Psychology* [2019] 10:1818).

Introduction

This chapter builds on attachment theory (Bowlby, 1969; Holmes, 1993, 1994; Main, 2000; Holmes & Slade, 2018) and draws on the links made between it and MUS as explained by Adshead and Guthrie (2015). Its contribution to knowledge lies in that it describes how TBMA, using a biopsychosocial model, can support people with MUS who also have insecure attachment. The rationale for the use of TBMA as opposed to other/psychological interventions is that the characteristics of insecure attachment are seen in people with MUS, so TBMA has been specifically designed in content and structure to work with these characteristics. It has been shown to be effective, in research, at reducing participant's symptoms, anxiety and depression and increasing wellbeing, activity levels and overall functioning (Payne & Stott, 2010; Payne & Brooks, 2016, 2017, 2018; Payne, 2017a). The research also employed qualitative data (participants comments, Payne & Brooks, 2020) to assess the outcomes in an NHS community setting (Payne, 2014, 2017b). The concept here is that the effectiveness seen in the empirical research derives from the design (explained below in detail) of this novel approach which specifically addresses attachment-related issues for people suffering MUS. TBMA uses a learning methodology with the aim of self-managing symptoms (Payne & Brooks, 2020) rather than offering psychological treatment. We interpret self-management as an outcome due to the fact participants report seeking less external help for symptoms such as visiting general practitioners (GPs), the hospital and/or accident and emergency (A&E) departments. Therefore, TBMA provides a new, different and acceptable pathway for people with MUS and adds to the discourse and understanding of the condition and its management.

Attachment

Attachment is the social connection that a child forms with a primary caregiver for emotional support/ regulation (Munselland et al., 2012). Attachment

DOI: 10.4324/9781003460749-8

happens during a "critical period" between 6 and 24 months enabling the child to create a working blueprint for future relationships. This forms a pattern for the adult dependent on those from whom they seek and receive care (Bowlby, 1969), particularly relevant for people suffering MUS. Attachment style is embodied and to a large extent stored in implicit memory (Schachner, Shaver & Mikulincer, 2005; Bentzen, 2015).

When there is a perceived threat (real/imagined) to survival, wellbeing or safety, attachment behaviour kicks-in to reduce distress, for example, to increase proximity to, and receive soothing comfort/reassurance from, an identified attachment figure. Thereafter in the long term the adult has self-soothing behaviours for comfort when in distress, with a healthy pattern of self-care and trust in the adequacy of caregivers.

Medically Unexplained Symptoms

Medically unexplained symptoms (MUS) are common world-wide, affecting mostly women (Verhaak et al., 2006; Steinbrecher et al., 2011), young people and non-native speakers (Steinbrecher et al., 2011). Illness is the context from which their experience is constructed, hence people with MUS tend to overly-identify with their symptoms. Research has found people with MUS have increased social isolation (Dirkzwager & Verhaak, 2007), more functional impairments (Katon & Walker, 1998), andassociated depression (Mahli, Couston & Fizt, 2013), anxiety (Lowe et al., 2008) and poorer quality of life (Smith, Monson & Ray, 1986) when compared with non-MUS populations. Although moderate and severe MUS appear comorbidly with common mental disorders, a direct psychological causality to symptoms is too crude to explain most MUS (Henningsen, Zipfel & Hersog 2007).

One definition of MUS is chronic, persistent bodily symptoms for which no medical explanation has been found. MUS can also be termed "body distress disorder" (DSM-5, American Psychiatric Association 2022) or "somatic symptom disorder" (SSD) (DSM-5, American Psychiatric Association, 2013) within the mental health (MH) field, the latter defined as the total number of somatic symptoms and the degree to which the patient is concerned about them (both of which are the predictors of health outcome and use).

Of the ten most common symptoms (fatigue, chest pain, headache, dizziness, swelling, back pain, insomnia, shortness of breath, abdominal pain and numbness) GPs cannot find a medical explanation for 75% of them (Kroenke & Mangelsdorff, 1989). One in five GP consultations and 18% of consecutive attenders are for MUS (Taylor et al., 2012). Edwards et al. (2010) found studies from around the world showing MUS totals 26–35% in primary care and 50% in secondary care (Barsky & Borus, 1995).

Treatment studies have been varied with mixed outcomes. Most have been based on one single condition such as fibromyalgia, which has associated symptoms, although in practice patients have more than one additional condition. TBMA is different in that it can include all types of symptoms in one group. Schröder et al. (2012) is the only other study which found group cognitive behaviour therapy (CBT) to be effective with generic MUS conditions. TBMA is a group approach similar to those in CBT (Arnold, Speckens & Van Hermert, 2004; Zonneveld et al., 2012) and group psychotherapy (for example Selders et al., 2015). Treatments are normally found in specialised clinics and mental health centres, limiting accessibility as patients refuse mental health referrals (Raine et al., 2002; Allen & Woolfolk, 2010). Approaches derived from individual CBT reduce the strength and occurrence of symptoms and improve functioning (den Boeft et al., 2014). Short-term intensive dynamic psychotherapy reduces symptoms and visits to accident and emergency settings (Abbass et al., 2009). Mindfulness-based CBT may also be effective (van Ravesteijn et al., 2014). Training of GPs in reattribution therapy has had little success (Gask et al., 2011), however physical exercise (graded) and yoga have promising outcomes (Aamland, Werner, & Malterud, 2013; Yoshihara et al., 2014). None of these interventions mention insecure attachment patterns.

Attachment Issues

Not everyone has a secure attachment. Insecure attachment can derive from adverse child experiences (ACEs) such as neglect, emotional/physical/sexual abuse, separation, loss and trauma to create insecure future relationships (Murphy et al., 2014) into adulthood. This can result in vulnerability when managing stress, suppressing negative feelings and not caring for one's self. Trust in the carers' competence is eroded leading to withdrawal from help-seeking behaviour (Ciechanowski et al., 2002) which may be true for some MUS sufferers, dependent on the insecure attachment style involved. Insecure attachment may also result in difficulty to self-sooth (self-regulate) in adulthood during threat/stress.

Links between Insecure Attachment and Medically Unexplained Symptoms

Bodily symptoms may be felt as a threat to survival, wellbeing and safety, creating susceptibility to an insecure attachment pattern. Adshead and Guthrie (2015) reviewed the evidence that insecure attachment is common in people with MUS and with some long-term conditions. They found three studies relevant to insecure attachment style and MUS. For women in one health maintenance organisation (Ciechanowski et. al., 2002), only 34% had secure attachment, which was half the expected number for a non-clinical sample. The women exhibited fearful (21%), preoccupied (22%), and dismissing (23%) insecure attachment patterns. Furthermore, the number of symptoms reported were significantly associated with these patterns. A greater number of somatic symptoms were reported for preoccupied and fearful patterns compared with secure. Attendance costs/call outs were higher for people with insecure attachment patterns compared with secure ones. Patients presenting with MUS were 2.47 times more likely to have insecure attachment according to Taylor et al. (2000) and Taylor et al. (2012) who showed frequent attendance at GPs was related to insecure attachment style.

Waller et al. (2004) assessed attachment security in 37 patients with ICD-10 somatoform disorder (without severe physical or mental illness) compared with 20 healthy matched controls. Compared with 60% of controls, only 26% rated as securely attached. The healthy controls demonstrated the expected incidence of insecure attachment, that is 25% were dismissing and 15% were pre-occupied. Patients though had high levels of dismissing (48.6%) and pre-occupied (25.7%) attachment patterns in sharp contrast. Other studies showed how early insecure attachment patterns are more common in patients with MUS (Taylor at al., 2000; Ciechanowski et al., 2002; Spertus et al., 2003; Noyes et al., 2003). It is proposed here that symptoms could be related to threats to attachment and thus to the self, resulting in fragility.

Using natural stress adaptations such as flight, fight, freeze (for mobilisation), fold or faint (defensive immobilisation) does not appear to resolve the internal perceived threat to wellbeing, survival and safety presented by MUS because it is in the body and not the environment. There is a correlation between female survivors of sexual abuse and preoccupied or insecure attachment (Stalker & Davies, 1995). Additionally, ACEs and somatisation are linked (Waldinger et al., 2006), as are ACEs and attachment issues (Sansone, Wiederman & Sansone, 2001). Insecure attachment has also been linked to somatisation (Stuart & Noyes, 1999). Hence, ACEs are linked with both somatisation (of which MUS is a subset) and attachment issues.

We know from research that MUS is associated with cumulative ACEs, including attachment issues (Elbers et al., 2017). We know also that insecure attachment creates stress and stress can result in mental health conditions and/or MUS. Thus, it could be concluded, having unexplained bodily symptoms might be a way for people with some insecure attachment patterns to legitimately seek help to meet their physical needs from those expected to be unresponsive to emotional needs. Some insecure attachment patterns result in the perception that health professionals or carers are inadequate in reducing arousal levels to relieve stress. That is, the professional is experienced as the mirror of the early inadequate caregiver (i.e., the child's primary caregiver). Salmon et al. (2009) analysed patient communications with doctors suggesting a strong desire for emotional support from health professionals.

As MUS is often experienced as pain, we searched for studies highlighting pain in relation to attachment. A synthesis of empirical research examined the relationship between attachment and somatoform symptoms in 3,376 children and adolescents (Vesterling & Koglin, 2020). The reviewed studies distinguished between groups of secure and insecure attachment (Ainsworth

& Bell, 1970; Main & Solomon, 1986). The reviewed studies indicated a positive correlation between fearful attachment patterns and pain symptoms, while the latter correlated negatively with secure attachment style. Disorganised attachment style was linked to inflammatory markers rather than the avoidant and resistant attachment patterns. However, there were confounding variables which make the interpretation problematic; the correlation of insecure attachment patterns with inflammatory markers was stronger when combined with maternal depression, and attachment security was negatively correlated with child depression, which in turn correlated positively with disease severity. Significantly higher scores of anxiety, depression, and somatisation were observed in groups classified as ambivalently attached compared with groups classified as securely attached and avoidantly attached. One study found gender differences in the correlation between insecure attachment patterns and pain severity, it being stronger for females (Tremblay & Sullivan, 2010). In summary the analysis suggests that the relationship between insecure attachment patterns and somatic complaints may not be a superficial one (Vesterling & Koglin, 2020) but further research is needed. This review concluded that attachment patterns in MUS is an under explored area and research needs to clarify the nature of the relationship, the role of the confounding variables and the factors involved in the developmental path from ACEs to somatic complaints (Vesterling & Koglin, 2020). Research has shown the existence of attachment-somatic symptoms, a link between attachment and childhood trauma and a link between childhood trauma and somatic symptoms (Stuart & Noyes, 1999; Pietromonaco & Beck, 2019).

A systematic review by Greenman et al. (2024) showed that attachment mediates the relationship between traumatic childhood events and the onset of physical diseases such as diabetes and heart diseases. The review aimed to investigate the relationships among these three phenomena and the underlying mechanisms driving these associations. It included 11 articles which defined somatic symptoms following the DSM5 guidelines, i.e. somatic symptoms are any pathological condition, including both physical diseases with a clear physiological aetiology and somatic physical unexplained symptoms (American Psychiatric Association, 2013). The concept of emotion regulation is prevalent in this review in that the contribution of an insecure attachment style to the negative affect resulting from childhood traumatic experiences is manifested in ineffective distress regulation, which in turn posits a risk factor for health problems and difficulties in coping with somatic symptoms in adulthood (Greenman et al., 2024). Interventions need to acknowledge the role of attachment in chronic health conditions and go beyond cognitive behavioural therapy since attachment has a central role for stress-management in chronic conditions (Luyten & Van Houdenhove, 2013). This chimes with the importance of attachment for stress regulation in the management of MUS facilitated through the design of TBMA's programme and practices.

Brenk-Franz et al. (2017) found the positive patient–provider relationship moderated the impact of attachment on self-management. It has been found in Payne and Brooks (2016, 2020) that the participants valued the facilitator greatly. This relationship is key.

Waldinger et al. (2006) investigated whether insecure attachment mediates the relationship between childhood trauma and somatisation in adulthood. In 101 couples, childhood trauma was associated with increased levels of somatisation and insecure attachment, with different patterns for men and women. For women, insecure attachment fully mediated the relationship between childhood trauma and somatisation. However, for men, insecure attachment did not mediate this relationship; instead, both childhood trauma and insecure attachment independently contributed to their somatisation severity index scores. These findings indicate that, for men, both trauma and attachment are significant independent predictors of somatisation, whereas for women, childhood trauma influences somatisation indirectly through its impact on attachment (Waldinger et al., 2006). The observed gender differences may be attributed to the varying types of abuse experienced by men and women. Women were three times more likely to have experienced sexual abuse than men which profoundly affects attachment security, especially when the attachment figure is the perpetrator.

The onset and management of chronic health conditions such as migraine, chronic fatigue, cardiac illness, and lifetime MUS have been associated with insecure attachment patterns (Meredith & Strong, 2019), but further research is needed.

Hypotheses

Not everyone with insecure attachment will have MUS. However, Adshead and Guthrie (2015) showed three insecure attachment patterns associated with MUS: dismissing, pre- occupied and fearful, which are discussed below.

It has been demonstrated that TBMA is effective (Payne & Brooks, 2017) in promoting the self-management of symptoms. Building on the work of Adshead and Guthrie (2015), which demonstrates the link between MUS and some insecure attachment patterns, TBMA has been specifically designed to take account of different insecure attachment patterns. MUS presents as many and various symptoms. TBMA groups reflect this as they are heterogeneous. As a result, there will be some participants with insecure attachment as an underlying issue within these groups. At every stage, therefore, TBMA addresses issues of insecure attachment in the structure of the programme, facilitation, group content/practices and mind-set of the population. Rather than one-to-one models, or non-interactive class-based methods, such as dance, Tai Chi or yoga, TBMA is a group interactive model. It supports people with MUS to take the risk of interacting with others (facilitator and other group members) within a safe, regulated environment. It may be that this interaction is the element of TBMA which helps address insecure attachment patterns.

We hypothesise, in accounting for the effectiveness of TBMA, that it can address insecure attachment patterns, which may be present in some MUS sufferers, leading to their capacity to self-manage. There are considerable benefits from TBMA as a specific type of bodymind approach that differs in that it is a group approach that avoids the stigma of, or aversion to, psychological therapies. In TBMA people learn to live well by self-managing symptoms. All this makes TBMA different from somatic therapies such as somatic experiencing (Levine, 2015; Levine, Blakeslee & Sylvae, 2018), sensorimotor therapy (Ogden, 2006) and other contemporary body and mind approaches to trauma. Whilst people report TBMA has helped them with their symptoms, TBMA does not aim to transform trauma, relieve symptoms, help clients to discover the emotional and physical source of their trauma or discharge the consequences of that trauma from the nervous system. However, it does appear to support their ability to self-regulate/self-manage symptoms. Therefore, TBMA is unlike these models or any other psychological intervention.

The design of the model is apt for people with MUS because it is accessible and acceptable as a perceptual learning methodology rather than a psychological treatment intervention. This population often does not accept or understand psychological methods due to their physical experience and explanatory perception. Consequently, TBMA can engage this hard-to-reach population. It is also appropriate for people with MUS who additionally have insecure attachment because of the way in which it has been designed, described below.

It is hypothesised here that the pain from ACEs, e.g. emotional deprivation, is transported into the body unconsciously and held there as a bodily memory (Koch, Fuchs & Summa, 2012; Giuseppe, 2018) only to be triggered in response to stressful situations (van der Kolk, 2015). Furthermore, it is proposed here that the chronic stress of an insecure attachment style mediates emotional dysregulation which in turn could produce symptoms in the body.

The Three Insecure Adult Attachment Patterns

Consequently, the three insecure adult attachment patterns linked to MUS to which TBMA attends are: dismissing and pre-occupied (Bartholomew & Horowitz, 1991; Main, 2000); and fearful (Bartholomew & Horowitz, 1991). Not all participants attending TBMA groups will necessarily be insecurely attached, however the programme supports this population specifically and can be helpful to all.

Dismissing

There may be an expectation that inadequate attention or care from others will be received with a "dismissing" type of attachment style. There may be anxiety about their symptoms and fear they will not be believed or taken seriously by health professionals. There may also be anxiety so health professionals may assume there is a mental health condition. Therefore, any form of mental health referral is often rejected and generally the health service is seen as unhelpful. The GP and other health care providers may become, to the patient, "the inadequate carer" as they attract the patient's dismissive attitude.

Pre-occupied

In contrast, an individual with a "pre-occupied" attachment style could become more concerned about losing the relationship with a health care professional after tests and scans etc. are over, and/or treatment is not indicated. There may be anxiety this relationship will need to end; they may become overly needy and dependent, pre-occupied with the relationship through their symptoms, and so return to the GP frequently. Bodily symptoms engage both parties, the patient visiting the GP with more and more symptoms and becoming emotionally needy. The GP tries to find a resolution, so sends them again for more tests and scans etc., thus feeding their anxiety. These patients may be referred to by GPs as "frequent flyers".

Fearful

Waldinger et al. (2006) showed that fearful insecure attachment style is correlated with childhood trauma/ACEs and adult somatisation in women. When a child is abused/neglected by a significant, yet unreliable adult caregiver, fearful attachment ensues. In this style a self-image may develop whereby the child feels unworthy of support from others, and of caregivers as being unreliable, or damaging. The combination of caregiver/GP and patient experience in the consultation may develop frustration and misunderstandings. Consequently, there may be a poor GP–patient relationship, and reduced care. The patient may feel they might drive others away and/or trigger inadequate outcomes due to their emotional neediness. Furthermore, this may develop into a compensatory emphasis on care-seeking for unexplained symptoms, due to an increased attention to bodily sensations.

The BodyMind Approach

We propose the insecure attachment patterns above affect the sufferers' ability to self-manage, hence the need to develop a more secure attachment as part of learning to self-manage. TBMA is effective for supporting people with MUS

(Payne & Stott, 2010; Payne & Brooks, 2016, 2017, 2018) and we suggest this results from increasingly secure attachment patterns during the group process, enabling – in some participants – the development of self-management. Due to TBMA's purpose-built design (discussed in detail below) insecure attachment patterns may be re-worked. In our experience, working with the symptoms through the body using improvisation, movement play, clay modelling, collage, mark-making, bodymindfulness, creativity and body-mind-emotion connections enable participants to explore and access meaning (Kossak, 2009). Using the imagination and creativity in movement, for example, can tap into sensory-emotional connections allowing embodied tacit knowledge of the symptom (which may otherwise be inaccessible) to surface. In contrast to CBT, TBMA uses the notion of the embodied unconscious (van der Kolk, 2015) by accessing the sensory experience in the body acquired through lived experience of the symptom. Accessing meaning explicitly invites people to make their own interpretations of the symptoms, for example, describing how they feel about their symptom when making marks or moving hands. This symbolises for themselves their unconscious meaning to the symptom which helps to make their previously unconscious implicit experience explicit, which is similar to the way arts therapies work. However, the authors are unaware of any arts therapies being employed for supporting people with MUS to self-manage. Establishing meaning helps the participant to validate the symptom. This is liberating because many MUS sufferers have been disbelieved.

The embodied style of attachment may be symbolised by the relationship to the symptom and the facilitator. Cognitive behaviour therapy comes at the world from thinking about thinking (meta-cognition), i.e. content. TBMA, in contrast, when employing bodymindfulness comes at the world from the awareness of awareness (meta-witness of the experience of sensation and process). The ability to have awareness of awareness enables people to recognise the possibility of non-attachment to the symptom (Wallin, 2017).

Adshead and Guthrie (2015) propose mindfulness-based practices may help with MUS by improving regulation of negative affect and to alter the awareness of, and relationship to, pain and bodily experience. Additionally, they suggest approaches offering "here and now" bodily experience connecting with images, whereby links can emerge between physical sensations, emotions and relationships, also improving regulation of negative affect. They go on to recommend that "clinicians need to develop interventions that 'fit' the attachment narratives of individual patients, rather than forcing patients into one size fits all psychological therapeutic techniques" (Adshead and Guthrie, 2015, p. 8). TBMA satisfies this recommendation because it has been specifically designed to fit the attachment narratives of individuals in a group setting. All TBMA practices whist conducted in a group setting can engage individuals with their own individual bodily experiences and imagination. People are invited to explore their relationship with symptoms mindfully to improve self-regulation and change their relationship to their body and symptoms. Furthermore, TBMA works with the imagin-ation, bodily experiences and somatic mindfulness practices to help people make connections between emotions, sensations and relationships. TBMA works in the "present moment" to raise and change awareness of the bodily sensation and the individual's relationship to it (Payne, 2019). TBMA is framed as experiential learning (Kolb, 1984; Payne & Brooks, 2020) as well as transformative in adult learning (Payne, 2019). The exercises enable access to perceptions of symptoms through the facilitator coaching enactive and embodied mindful practices. They aim to shift the experience of the symptom, changing the relationship, perception and mind-set toward the symptom. This leads to the cultivation of self-management of symptoms thereby encouraging wellbeing.

Unlike psychological interventions in TBMA the body is emphasised first and foremost in deep connection, not as separate parts, hence written as "BodyMind", joined together, rather than "mind-body" with mind first and separated from body with a hyphen. TBMA works from the subjective body experience to the mind and back again. It privileges the interactive relationship between the body and mind, which is so emphasised in MUS. It focuses holistically on the whole person rather than relying solely on language with more of an emphasis on the right side of the brain (creative side). In TBMA there is no explicit discussion of psychological or causal relationship with the symptoms unless the participant makes such connec-tions themselves.

The BodyMind Approach transforms seeing symptoms or the body as the "enemy" in a dismissive attachment style to embracing them as an "ally", flagging up the need for self-care and compassionate acceptance of symptoms/self (Payne & Brooks, 2018; 2019, 2020). Caring for the self (self-soothing normally developed from early attachment experiences) is ini-tially modelled by the facilitator as a proxy caregiver, e.g. their explain-ing how to sit, breathe, use bodymindfullness and listen to the body for signs of stress. Practices compare symptom sensations with other areas of the body as functioning and positive to create a balance between health and "dys-ease". Rather than immobility, as in mindfulness, TBMA encourages mindful mobility/mindful movement which favours agency, and somatic mindfulness, for example, "being in the movement moment" as in walking around the space together with a focus on the visceral experience of what is happening in the body and to the symptom in action. In common with trauma approaches (Ogden, 2006) the vital aspect of mobilisation, which favours agency, is recognised. This contrasts with CBT in which agency is contemplated and planned for in the future rather than experiencing agency in the present practice.

Group interaction is important to aid different patterns of attachment with peers rather than solely with the facilitator, who for some may be seen as a health professional to whom they may have a corresponding negative attitude (dismissive style), although this attitude may not be so prominent with the group members. The group gives the opportunity for shared resources. A sense of belonging helps engagement, reduces isolation and promotes "happy" hormones – for example dopamine, oxytocin, serotonin and endorphins – to be released (Porges, 2003; van der Kolk, 2015).

Three Key Concepts

The BodyMind Approach® is designed to support people with MUS and insecure attachment to learn to self-manage through three key concepts pragmatically built into the programme.

a) Emotional regulation
b) Safety
c) Bodymindfulness

a) Emotional regulation

Emotional regulation is how a person manages feelings with cognitive, physiological and behavioural associated processes. It is the process that raises or lowers the degree of emotions (Parrott, 1993) to enhance well-being. This emotional self-regulation framework provides for vitality but also reduced arousal for calmness. It is developed through attunement with a reliable caregiver. Attachment is therefore a significant aspect of emotional self-regulation. More securely attached children rate higher in emotional regulation and empathy (Panfile & Laible, 2012) and TBMA appears to overcome the powerful blueprint of early insecure attachment patterns, using the relationship with the facilitator and the group to cultivate a more secure relationship enabling the development of resilience drawing on neuroplasticity.

Holmes (1993) reporting on Bowlby indicates that attachment is a primary motivational system related to a spatial environment in association with a loved one. When an individual feels safe and securely attached to the loved one, they can begin to pursue exploration. When they feel unsafe, dysregulated signs of distress appear in their behaviour. TBMA engages with individuals to explore their symptoms by providing a safe external environment. The facilitator models unconditional positive regard and a non-judgemental attitude. When this is combined with stable, closed, group membership (with few withdrawals), a constant space, predicted dates/times for meetings and a consistent facilitator, safety ensues making for regulated behaviour.

b) The importance of safety in groups

Participants were requested to commit to the first six sessions and thereafter for the following six. The opportunity to withdraw after the first six sessions appeared to add to the safety element for some people but was never used. Paradoxically, it seems likely that this structure was less threatening for individuals with a fearful or dismissive style, enabling them to complete the 12 sessions. Participants with a pre-occupied style would feel compelled to complete anyway.

In Maslow's (1943) hierarchy of needs for self-actualisation the first is physiological, then comes safety needs followed by the need for a sense of belonging. Insecure attachment means that a sense of belonging is missing, maybe because social engagement is too difficult. We know reliable safety is crucial to allow social engagement to occur. When safety and wellbeing is threatened, as in MUS, there is a greater need for safety to reduce the activation of the stress adaption response of mobility (Porges, 2018). In people with both MUS and insecure attachment, the need for safety is even more critical. Hence the group needs to be a safe place – non-threatening and social – to give a sense of belonging through the shared purpose. Another aspect of safety in TBMA sessions is that no one need disclose their symptom/s, which helps enable experimentation and exploration of symptoms.

c) *Bodymindfulness*

Depression and/or anxiety often accompany MUS (Rosmalen & de Jonge, 2010; Burton et al., 2011). Mindfulness reduces depression and anxiety (Hofmann et al., 2010) and has a moderate effect on some MUS, such as pain (Grossman et al., 2004). Segal, Williams and Teasdale (2002) found an association between a lack of mindful self-awareness and depression, resulting in poor recognition of and reflection on bodily cues or signals like tension, pain and fatigue. A "mindful attitude" can be defined as a state of presence moment to moment, realised through intentionally directed attention. At the same time both internal body sensations and external stimuli can enter and leave awareness without judgment. For example, kindly attending to the symptom sensation interoceptively can, ironically, reduce the distress experienced. A mindful state results from participating in the state as though one was an empathic witness "benignly regarding the self".

"Bodymindfulness" incorporates body awareness practices and movement in the present moment ("kinaesthetic mindfulness"). Employing these two practices enables the relationship with the symptom to be explored and understood. It can help with dis-identification with bodily symptoms which is so often tied up with identity for the individual with MUS (Sanders, Winter & Payne, 2018).

The Design of TBMA to Support Insecure Attachment

TBMA intervention is referred to as "learning groups", "symptoms groups" and/or "workshops" to GPs and patients, with a focus on the lived body experience of the symptoms rather than any mental health or psychological title. People in the groups are referred to as "participants" rather than "patients" which may help a sense of agency since it reduces dependency and any expectations the facilitator will be unsatisfactory. The programme normalises the symptoms, i.e. non-medicalising them, which helps acceptance of the condition and promotes feelings of agency, where previously there may have been none. For all insecure attachment patterns this sense of agency can be helpful for engagement.

The group workshops are held twice a week for the first two weeks. This intensity at the outset helps to promote cohesiveness in the group. Bonds can be forged with each other and the facilitator, promoting engagement and reducing drop-out. The 12 x 2 hourly sessions are optimal for change (Lambert, 2013) with enough time for engagement. The individual consultation with the facilitator, conducted before the group commences and the week it ends, is in the same venue as the group sessions, which can add reassurance for individuals with pre-occupied attachment patterns. Participants are aware they will be contacted by the facilitator every six weeks for a further six months, i.e. they are not dropped after the group ends. A participant who has a pre-occupied attachment style will be reassured by the level of contact on-going; initially the fearfully attached will be frightened but they can opt in or out after six sessions or 12. The dismissive insecure attachment style participant will disengage and attempt to sabotage the group. However, the facilitator having a very high level of psychological skills can "hold" the group and provide enough safety to prevent disintegration occurring.

Even though the origin of somatic symptoms may be found in developmental trauma (i.e. insecure attachment patterns), in TBMA the formulation for practice is in the biopsychosocial response rather than in a psychotherapeutic one.

The sessions are carefully structured to cultivate interaction with rituals and predictable events for safety which support the fearful and preoccupied insecure attachment patterns substantially. There is predictable on-going contact between participants and facilitators, even after face-to-face contact has concluded, via the six-weekly texts, emails and/or letters. This seems to reduce concerns whether participants have fearful, dismissing or a pre-occupied attachment style.

The Power of the Group

For people with MUS who are insecurely attached the group can act as a support and pathway towards learning to make healthy attachments in a safe setting. The group acts as a source of peer support rather than support being from one health professional, i.e. from only the therapist/teacher as in one-to-one approaches. Friendships test out and strengthen the ability to form more secure attachments. Group solidarity and approbation develop, encouraging each other towards improvement. The group shares goals, for example, improving health and wellbeing and the belief in hope for change. These shared goals/beliefs help form the group identity, rationale for the sense of belonging, the protection offered and the group's continuous existence through the bond created (Bar-Tal, 2000). This type of group for this population which has tended to experience isolation can be a welcome "comfort blanket", bridging them into a different world of experimentation and exploration.

The group gives permission to share intimate personal stories. Participants discover common experiences shared in the group, they feel less isolated, make friends and often meet up following the group. The fact people wish to meet after the group is in line with group identification and group attachment. Smith, Murphy and Coats (1999) explain how the subsystems and functions regulating one-to-one attachment are the same as attachment to social groups. These include seeking support and responsiveness and emotional disclosure, all of which are affected by personal history, which in turn affects future relationships. Bearing this in mind, careful preparation is given to the beginning and ending of sessions and to the whole programme. For example, cohesion is strongly encouraged, and safety promoted from the outset. Additionally, there are individual consultations with the facilitator, an action plan for going forward post-group and non-face-to-face contact every six weeks for six months. The group's capacity to act as an attachment object and provider of security can affect neural integration. The group may help to down-regulate participants' emotions by being a regular, steady influence in their lives. Porges' Polyvagal Theory (Porges, 2003) concludes that human social interaction combined with taking the psychological mind-set into account in interventions turns off the sympathetic fight/flight response. The calming of the sympathetic nervous system, combined with feeling listened to, enables people to feel safe enough to engage in the play. This enables the work of self-reflection, self-regulation and self-management (Porges, 2003).

It is possible that the group may be self-selecting since people who tend to avoid attachment or who are anxiously attached may filter themselves out before committing. Anxiously attached participants may be frightened of rejection so might be overly positive of their experiences.

The Facilitator as a Catalyst

Bowlby (1969, p. 207) suggests "the link between leader and group is a facilitating, rather than a necessary element of the individual's attachment to the group". Nevertheless, Sochos (2015) claims there can be an attachment to the group via an internalised, individual image which symbolises the group. He goes on to say there is a sense of security and protection derived from the leader – a powerful other – and hence in TBMA the attachment is both with the facilitator and the group as a whole.

The facilitator initially holds the hope for the group and that change is possible. This helps transform the group mind-set to a more positive one. Facilitators have a passion for the approach which influences engagement from the group. They are all trained and certified in the facilitation of TBMA groups, have experience of over five years in leading groups of adults in mental health and a background in embodied, enactive approaches. Furthermore, facilitators are selected based on their qualities of warmth, empathy and genuineness (Rogers, 1961). The facilitator's training and attitudes are specifically geared towards supporting individuals with insecure attachment.

The individual consultation with the group facilitator at the outset sets the tone for the group workshops, building early rapport with the group facilitator to provide safety. An insecurely attached participant will have opportunities to see and experience secure attached relationships and to transform their relationship with the facilitator over time. This early relationship set up may help calm anxieties and helps to ensure future participation and relationship formation.

The individual consultation with the facilitator at the end of the group helps reflection, closure, clarification of their action plan for self-management and support arranged for this during the following six months. This consultation and the last group session provide for preparation for the ending of the group which is so important for pe-occupied insecurely attached participants who will not have had many experiences of good-enough endings. The subsequent six months of non-face-to-face contact with the facilitator supports continuity, a sense of agency to self-manage and the embedment of new habits promoted via their action plan.

Each insecure attachment style has its own characteristics, and we speculate below on how these are interacted with through the design of structure, facilitation and practices of TBMA intervention.

Dismissive

In this style there is a positive view of self (I am ok) and a negative view of others (you are not ok). A dismissing type of attachment style may bring the expectation of inadequate attention or care that will be received from others. Those who care for them, such as GPs, are not OK. In TBMA, people are in a group with shared experiences of the health service which may, perhaps, reinforce their lived experience of inadequate care. However, the other participants are not their carers/health professionals (nor authority figures) and this is an important advantage for their sources of support. People share their experience, strengths and hopes for change. This is empowering. Participants are encouraged to consider ways to care for themselves (self-sooth), manage stress levels and re-interpret their symptom distress.

This individual usually rejects any form of mental health referral and generally sees the health service as unhelpful for their MUS. In order to facilitate acceptance and access for this style, TBMA is framed as "workshops" for "self-management" rather than a medical intervention or mental health treatment methodology.

People with a dismissive style deny and minimise the impact of their own experience and their feelings. They tend to lack confidence in helpers and in their ability to help themselves. They may have poor self-reflection and tend to be critical of practices and helpers to date (e.g. GP). In order to accommodate this the facilitator accepts and welcomes their stance non-judgementally and reflects it back to the participant to support and validate it. This avoids criticism of the helper. Other group members then act as models for reflection, again taking the attention away from the facilitator. The facilitator encourages mobilisation to generate more experience on which to reflect and to think about the meaning of their symptom.

Pre-occupied

In the pre-occupied style people tend to feel overwhelmed by their symptoms. The stance taken by the facilitator is that many people have unexplained symptoms which she can work with, thus normalising the condition and reducing fear. There is also the threat of what will happen if they lose their symptoms, i.e. a leap of faith into the unknown. Eventually, after a while, when trust has been established this can be addressed by exploring the pros and cons of having the symptom. The facilitator forms a stable attachment figure, as does the group, thus engendering trust. The nonverbal communication of the body is a root to access what is, as yet, unknown regarding the meaning of the symptom. So, practices employing movement such as gestures and postures to represent the sensation of the symptom may bring meaning to the forefront and in-depth knowing which cannot be arrived at in any other way.

In the pre-occupied attachment style, there is a negative model of self, a positive model of others – "I am not OK, others are OK". The pre-determined frequency and nature of the contact post-group is reassuring for people with a pre-occupied attachment style. The facilitator models self-acceptance and compassion, enabling people to develop a more solid, coherent sense of self and to acknowledge their own vulnerabilities resulting from their experiences.

Additionally, the attachment may be more secure as a result of the programme, enabling them to become less dependent on the GP – as the monitoring of the six-month follow up showed (Payne & Brooks, 2016). This participant may find the ending of the group problematic and experience it as loss. The closing exit consultation meeting with the facilitator mitigates some of this but also groups do tend to go on meeting following the ending. Another strategy to support the pre-occupied participant is the on-going non-face-to-face contact every six weeks post-group. The shared decision making (with the facilitator) of their tailor-made action plan (derived from experiences and new understanding to support new habits of self-management) also helps with the ending process and sustainability.

The efficacy of TBMA in promoting self-management enables participants who have a pre-occupied insecure attachment style to accept their condition, obviating the need for further tests and scans for their symptom/s. TBMA promotes a belief they can live well and thrive despite their symptoms. Their symptom distress levels and anxiety decrease as they let go of the need for a medical explanation.

Fearful

Individuals who are fearfully attached have a negative model of self and others – "neither are OK". They may present as angry, frustrated and difficult, and are prone to develop a self-image as unworthy of support from others and an image of caregivers as unreliable, or even dangerous. TBMA's programme promotes a sense of agency and self-care, i.e. one is deserving of care for themselves. The facilitator understands the importance of always being present for the group by demonstrating reliability, which in turn offers safety. Both participants with fearful insecure attachments and the facilitator may experience misunderstanding and frustration. However, regular supervision supports the facilitator to contain any frustrations and to ensure best practice when working with these participants.

People with a fearful attachment style may worry about not being believed and taken seriously by health care providers who may assume they have a mental health condition. In TBMA the participant's lived body experience is believed and symptoms honoured. They also worry about their symptoms which defy diagnosis, despite numerous investigations, tests and scans which can lead to catastrophising about them. The embodied, pre-verbal feelings, thoughts and impulses from an attachment style laid down in early attachment may be repeated symbolically in the participant's relationship to their symptom. In the TBMA group people are helped to change their stance towards their experience of the symptom through a shift in the view of self. This may be a dynamic relationship with the symptom and the self. The view of self becomes much more than simply the symptom, thus reducing the tendency to catastrophise.

The participant may sense their emotional neediness may drive others away. Emotional needs are welcome in the group, although the facilitator ensures shared attention is available to each member. People who are fearfully attached may avoid long-term care situations because of concerns about greater intimacy with providers and an assumption they will be given insufficient care. Hence TBMA is short term: the number of sessions overall is 12, the first four are in the first two weeks (i.e. two sessions per week), of two hours duration each, with an opt-out after session six. Twelve sessions are the optimum for engagement for group psychotherapy according to Lambert (2013).

Fears about caregiver dependability promotes GP-shopping, i.e. visiting each GP in a practice and/or changing practices frequently, and a fragmentation of care. For TBMA groups there are a number of participants to offer resources and care. The caregiver-facilitator may experience people who are fearfully attached as difficult to reassure, inadequate, needy and fragile. Facilitators are trained to expect participants like this and have strategies to support them, e.g. offering alternatives to practices, treating the practices as experiments to try out – reducing risk and stakes, lessening exposure.

Individual consultations with the facilitator before the group sessions provide an opportunity for this participant to ask questions and gain reassurance leading to feelings of safety. This mediates the initial stress of attending a group of unknown people.

The outreach of six months non-face-to-face contact subsequent to the group ending can feel safer than being in the group whilst maintaining an on-going relationship with the group facilitator. This can replace seeking care in settings such as accident and emergency. The TBMA programme is designed to support participants over a period of nine months. It has been found that the 12 face-to-face sessions over ten weeks in the first three months are just about manageable and bearable for the fearfully insecurely attached participant.

Summary

The empirical research conducted previously supports the hypothesis that TBMA can support people with insecure attachment patterns and MUS to self-manage. This article has illustrated how the design of TBMA is built on the three adult insecure attachment patterns associated with MUS. It goes on to explain how TBMA helps people with MUS and insecure attachment patterns to learn to self-manage. Its contribution to knowledge lies in that it describes a novel group model (TBMA) designed specifically as a new alternative pathway for supporting people with MUS to self-manage, some of whom may be insecurely attached. The programme is particularly suited as an intervention for people with MUS because symptoms are experienced in the body first and foremost. In TBMA groups those symptoms are honoured, using them as a gateway to the mind and subsequent self-management, in contrast to CBT which tends to marginalise the body. The TBMA model is also different because it can include people with all sorts of conditions in a generic group.

Early attachment is first experienced through the body via touch from the primary caregiver (White, 2004). Body memory (Giuseppe, 2018) of early attachment is reflected in relationships in the future, including the relationship with the symptom which can become a metaphor for the individual's insecure attachment. The TBMA groups work with the symptom and its meaning employing the body-felt sensation of the symptom as the basis for learning self-management. It seems likely that the pain from adverse child-hood experiences is transported into the body unconsciously and held there as a bodily memory only to be triggered in response to stressful situations to form an MUS. By learning to acknowledge and address the stress, MUS suffering can be self-managed (Lind, Delmar & Nielsen, 2014).

The programme for TBMA is innovative since all elements involved have been designed to compensate for insecure attachment issues. This includes programme structure, qualities of facilitation, group methods and content accounting for safety, self-regulation and bodymindfulness. The group and facilitator are crucial to outcomes for participants, helping to prevent the repetition of dysfunctional attachment patterns affecting the maintenance of self-management to sustain recovery. In TBMA a re-sculpting of the self and the symptom and their relationship to each other is enabled. The improved self-management participants, when tested for effectiveness through rigorous practice-based research, exhibited reduced symptom distress, depression and anxiety, and increased wellbeing, activity and overall functioning (Payne & Brooks 2016; 2017). It is proposed the behaviour changes noted have become conscious, which is essential for self-management. Importantly, there are also potential reduced costs for the health service and in GP time and resources (Payne, 2014).

The hypothesis that TBMA can address insecure attachment in people with MUS can be tested in the framework of current knowledge by conducting an adult attachment assessment (Bartholomew & Shaver, 1998) pre- and post-intervention with participants suffering MUS and undergoing TBMA treatment.

References

Aamland, A., Werner, E. L., and Malterud, K. (2013). Sickness absence, marginality, and medically unexplained physical symptoms: a focus-group study of patients' experiences. *Scandinavia Journal of Primary Health Care*, Jun; 31(2), 95–100. doi: 10.3109/02813432.2013.788274.

Abbass, A., Campbell, S., Magee, K et al. (2009). Intensive short-term dynamic psychotherapy to reduce rates of emergency department return visits for patients with medically unexplained symptoms: preliminary evidence from a pre-post intervention study. *CJEM*, Nov; 11(6), 529–534.

Adshead, G. and Guthrie, E. (2015). The role of attachment in medically unexplained symptoms and long-term illness. *British Journal of Psychological Advances*, (21)3, 167–174.

Ainsworth, M. D. S., and Bell, S.M. (1970). Attachment, exploration, and separation: illustrated by the behavior of one-year-olds in a strange situation, *Child Dev*, 41, 49–67.

Allen, L. A. and Woolfolk, R. L. (2010). Cognitive behavioral therapy for somatoform disorders. *Psychiatric Clinics of North America*, 33, 579–593.

American Psychiatric Association. (2013). *Diagnostic and Statistical Manual of Mental Disorders-5*. American Psychiatric Association.

Arnold, I. A., Speckens, A. E. M., and Van Hermert, A. M. (2004). Medically unexplained physical symptoms: the feasibility of group cognitive-behavioural therapy in primary care. *Journal of Psychosomatic Research*, 57: 517–520.

Barsky, A. J., and Borus, J. F. (1995). Somatization and medicalization in the era of managed care. *JAMA*, 274(24), 1931–1934.

Bar-Tal, D. (2000). *Shared Beliefs in a Society: Social Psychological Analysis*. Sage.

Bartholomew, K. and Horowitz, L. M. (1991). Attachment styles among young adults: a test of a four-category model. *Journal of Personality and Social Psychology*, 61, 2, 226–244.

Bartholomew, K., and Shaver, P. R. (1998). Methods of assessing adult attachment: Do they converge? In J. A. Simpson and W. S. Rholes (Eds), *Attachment Theory and Close Relationships* (pp. 25–45). The Guilford Press.

Bentzen, M. (2015). Dances of connection: Neuro-affective development in clinical work with attachment. *Body Movement and Dance in Psychotherapy*, 10(4), 211–226, 10.1080/17432979.2015.1064479

Bowlby, J. (1969). *Attachment and Loss, Volume 1*. Basic Books.

Brenk-Franz, K., Srauß, B., ... and Gensichen, J. (2017). Patient–provider relationship as mediator between adult attachment and self-management in primary care patients with multiple conditions. *J. Psychosom. Res.*, 97, 131–135.

Burton, C., McGorm, K., Weller, D., and Sharpe, M. (2011). Depression and anxiety in patients repeatedly referred to secondary care with medically unexplained symptoms: a case-control study. *Psychological Medicine*, 41(3), 555–563. Epub 2011/ 01/29. pmid:21272387

Ciechanowski, P. S., Walker, E. A., Katon, W. J., and Russo, J. E. (2002). Attachment theory: A model for health care utilization and somatization. *Psychosomatic Medicine*, 64, 660–667.

Den Boeft, M., van der Wouden, J. C. ... and Numans, M. E. (2014). Identifying patients with medically unexplained physical symptoms in electronic medical records in primary care: a validation study. *BMC Family Practice*, Jun 515(1), 109. doi: 10.1186/1471-2296-15-109.

Dirkzwager, A. J. E., and Verhaak, P. F. M. (2007). Patients with persistent medically unexplained symptoms in general practice: characteristics and quality of care. *BMC Family Practice*, 8(33), https://doi.org/10.1186/1471-2296-8-33

Edwards, T. M., Stern, A., ... and Kasney, L. M. (2010). The treatment of patients with medically unexplained symptoms in primary care: A review of the literature. *Mental Health Family Medicine*, Dec7 (4), 209–221.

Elbers, J., Rovnaghi, C. R., Golianu, B. and, Anand, K. J. S. (2017). Clinical Profile Associated with Adverse Childhood Experiences: The Advent of Nervous System Dysregulation. Children (Basel). *Children*, 4(11), 98. doi:10.3390/children4110098

Gask, L., Dowrick, C., ... and Morriss, R. (2011) Reattribution reconsidered: narrative review and reflections on an educational intervention for medically unexplained symptoms in primary care settings. *Psychosomatic Research*, Nov71(5), 325–334. doi: 10.1016/j.jpsychores.2011.05.008.

Giuseppe, R. (2018). The neuroscience of body memory: From the self through the space to the others. *Cortex*, 104, 241–260.

Greenman, P. S., Renzi, A. ... and Di Trani, M. (2024). How does trauma make you sick? The role of attachment in explaining somatic symptoms of survivors of childhood trauma. *Healthcare 12*, 203. https://doi.org/10.3390/healthcare1 2020203

Grossman, P., Niemann, L., Schmidt, S., and Walach, H. (2004). Mindfulness-based stress reduction and health benefits. A meta-analysis. *Psychosomatic Research.* Jul; 57(1), 35–43.

Henningsen, P., Zipfel, S., and Herzog, W. (2007). Management of functional somatic syndromes. *Lancet*, 369(9565), 946–955.

Hofmann, S. G., Sawyer, A. T., Witt, A. A., and Oh, D. (2010). The effect of mindfulness-based therapy on anxiety and depression: A meta-analytic review. *Consult Clinical Psychology*, Apr; 78(2), 169–183. doi: 10.1037/a0018555

Holmes, J. (1993). *John Bowlby and Attachment Theory.* Routledge. doi:10.4324/ 9780203136805

Holmes, J. (1994). Attachment theory – a secure theoretical base for counselling? *Psychodynamic Counselling*, 1(1), 65–78, doi: 10.1080/13533339408404713

Holmes, J. and Slade, A. (2018). *Attachment in Therapeutic Practice.* Sage.

Katon, W. J. and Walker, E. A. (1998). Medically unexplained symptoms in primary care. *Clin. Psychiatry*, 59, 15–21.

Koch, S., Fuchs, T and Summa, M. (2012). *Body Memory, Metaphor and Movement.* John Benjamins Publishing.

Kolb, D. A. (1984). Experiential learning: Experience as the source of learning and development. New Jersey: Prentice Hall.

Kossak, M. S. (2009). Therapeutic attunement: a transpersonal view of expressive arts therapy. *The Arts in Psychotherapy*, 36, 13–18.

Kroenke, K., and Mangelsdorff, A. D. (1989). Common symptoms in ambulatory care: incidence, evaluation, therapy and outcome. *Am. J. Medicine*, 86, 262–266.

Lambert, M. J. (2013). The efficacy and effectiveness of psychotherapy. In: A. E., Bergin and S. L., Garfield (Eds), *Handbook of Psychotherapy and Behaviour Change*, 6th edn (Chapter 6). John Wiley and Sons.

Levine, P (2015). *Trauma and Memory: Brain and Body in a Search for the Living Past: A Practical Guide for Understanding and Working with Traumatic Memory.* North Atlantic Books.

Levine, P. A., Blakeslee, A., and Sylvae, J. (2018). Reintegrating fragmentation of the primitive self: Discussion of "somatic experiencing". *Psychoanalytic Dialogues*, 28(5), 620–628.

Lind, A. B., Delmar, C., and Nielsen, K. (2014). Searching for existential security: a prospective qualitative study on the influence of mindfulness therapy on experienced stress and coping strategies among patients with somatoform disorders. *J. Psychosom. Res*, Dec; 77(6), 516–521. doi: 10.1016/j.jpsychores.2014.07.015

Lowe, B., Spitzer, R. L., ... and Kroenke, K. (2008). Depression, anxiety and somatization in primary care: Syndrome overlap and functional impairment. *General Hospital Psychiatry*, 30(3), 191–199.

Luyten, P., and Van Houdenhove, B. (2013). Common and specific factors in the psychotherapeutic treatment of patients suffering from chronic fatigue and pain. *J. Psychotherapy Integrative*, 23, 14–27.

Main, M., and Solomon, J. (1986). Discovery of an insecure-disorganized/disoriented attachment pattern. In: T. B. Brazelton and Yogman (Eds), *Affective Development in Infancy* (pp. 95–124). Ablex Publishing.

Main, M. (2000). The Adult Attachment Interview: Fear, attention, safety and discourse processes. *Journal of the American Psychoanalytic Association*, 48, 1055–1095.   https://attachmentdisorderhealing.com/adult-attachment-interview-aai-mary-main/

Malhi, G. S., Couston, C. M. and Fizt, K. (2013). Unlocking the diagnosis of depression in primary care: Which key symptoms are GPs using to determine diagnosis and severity? *Australian and New Zealand Journal of Psychiatry*, 48(6).

Maslow, A. H. (1943). A theory of human motivation. *Psychological Review*, 50(4), 370–396. doi:10.1037/h0054346

Meredith, P. J., and Strong, J. (2019). Attachment and chronic illness. *Current Opinion in Psychology*, 25, 132–138. https://doi.org/10.1016/j.copsyc.2018.04.018

Murphy, A., Steele, M. ... and Steele, H. (2014). Adverse Childhood Experiences (ACEs) questionnaire and Adult Attachment Interview (AAI): implications for parent child relationships. *Child Abuse Neglect*, 38, 224–233. doi: 10.1016/j.chiabu.2013.09.004

Munsell, E. P., Kilmer, R. P., Cook, J. R. and Reeve, C. L. (2012). The effects of caregiver social connections on caregiver, child, and family well-being. *Am. J. Orthopsychiatry*, Jan; 82(1), 137–145. doi: 10.1111/j.1939-0025.2011.01129.x

Noyes, R. J., Stuart, ... and Yagla, S. J. (2003). Test of an interpersonal model of hypochondriasis. *Psychosomatic Medicine*, Mar–Apr; 65(2), 292–300.

Ogden, P. (2006). *Trauma and the Body: A Sensorimotor Approach to Psychotherapy* (Norton Series on Interpersonal Neurobiology). Norton.

Panfile, T. M. and Laible, D. J. (2012). Attachment security and child's empathy: the mediating role of emotion regulation. *Merrill-Palmer Quarterly*, 58, 1, 1–21.

Parrott, W. G. (1993). Beyond hedonism: Motives for inhibiting good moods and for maintaining bad moods. In D. M. Wegner and J. W. Pennebaker (Eds), *Handbook of Mental Control* (pp. 278–305). Prentice Hall.

Payne, H. (2014) Patient experience: push past symptom mysteries. *Health Service J.*, 124(6390), 26–27.

Payne, H. (2017a) Reliable change in outcomes from The BodyMind Approach™ with people who have medically unexplained symptoms/somatic symptom disorder in primary healthcare. In: H. Payne (Ed.) *Essentials of Dance Movement Psychotherapy* (pp. 149–172). Routledge.

Payne, H. (2017b). Transferring research from a University into the National Health Service: implications for impact. *Health Research Systems and Policy*, Opinion Piece, 15(56) DOI 10.1186/s12961-017-0219-3.

Payne, H. (2019). The BodyMind Approach and people affected by medically unexplained symptoms/somatic symptom disorder. In H. Payne, S. Koch, J. Tantia (Eds) *The Routledge International Handbook of Embodied Perspectives in Psychotherapy* (pp. 195–203). Routledge.

Payne, H. and Brooks, S.D.M. (2016). Clinical outcomes from The BodyMind Approach in the treatment of patients with medically unexplained symptoms in primary healthcare in England: Practice-based evidence. *The Arts in Psychotherapy*, 47, 55–65.

Payne, H. and Brooks, S.D.M., (2017). Moving on: The BodyMind Approach for medically unexplained symptoms. *Public Mental Health* 10, 1–9. doi: 10.1108/JPMH-10-2016-0052

Payne, H. and Brooks, S. (2018). Different strokes for different folks: The BodyMind Approach as a learning tool for patients with medically unexplained symptoms to self-manage. *Front. Psychol.* 9, 2222. doi: 10.3389/fpsyg.2018.02222

Payne, H. and Brooks S.D. (2019). Medically Unexplained Symptoms and Attachment Theory: The BodyMind Approach. *Front Psychol.* Nov 6, 10, 1818. doi: 10.3389/fpsyg.2019.01818. PMID: 31780974; PMCID: PMC6851196.

Payne, H. and Brooks S.D.M. (2020). A qualitative study of the views of patients with Medically Unexplained Symptoms on The BodyMind Approach: employing embodied methods and arts practices for self-management. *Front. Psychol.*, 11, 554566. doi: 10.3389/fpsyg.2020.554566.

Payne, H., and Stott, D. (2010). Change in the moving bodymind: quantitative results from a pilot study on the use of the BodyMind Approach (BMA) to psychotherapeutic group work with patients with medically unexplained symptoms (MUSs). *Counselling and Psychotherapy Research*, 10(4), 295–306. https://doi.org/10.1080/14733140903551645

Pietromonaco, P. R. and Beck, L. A. (2019) Adult attachment and physical health. *Curr. Opin. Psychol.*, 25, 115–120.

Porges, S. (2003). Social engagement and attachment: a phylogenetic perspective. *Annals of New York Academy of Sciences*, 1008, 31–47.

Porges, S. (2018). *Clinical Applications of Polyvagal Theory: The Emergence of Polyvagal Informed Therapies.* W. W. Norton and Co.

Raine, R., Haines, A., Sensky, T., Hutchings, A., Larkin, K. et al. (2002). Systematic review of mental health interventions for patients with common somatic symptoms: can research evidence from secondary care be extrapolated to primary care? *British Medical Journal*, 325, 1082–1092.

Rogers, C. (1961). *On Becoming a Person.* Constable.

Rosmalen, J. G. M., and de Jonge, P. (2010). Empirical foundation for the diagnosis of somatization: implications for DSM-5. *Psychological Medicine*, 41, 1133–1142. pmid:2084340

Salmon, P., Ring, A., Humphris, G. M., Davies, J. C., and Dowrick, C. F. (2009). Primary care consultations about medically unexplained symptoms: how do patients indicate what they want? *Journal of General Internal Medicine*, 24, 450–456.

Sandel, S. L., Judge, J. O., Landry, N., Faria, L., Ouellette, R., and Majczak, M. (2005). Dance and movement program improve quality-of-life measures in breast cancer survivors. *Cancer Nursing*, 28, 4, 301–309.

Sanders, T., Winter, D., and Payne, H. (2018) Personal constructs of mind-body identity in people who experience medically unexplained symptoms. *Journal of Constructivist Psychology*, 32(4), 408–423. doi: 10.1080/10720537.2018.1515047

Sansone, R. A., Wiederman, M. and Sansone, L. (2001). Adult somatic preoccupation and its relationship to childhood trauma. *Violence and Victims*, 16, 39–47.

Schachner, P. R., Shaver, M., and. Mikulincer, M. (2005). Patterns of nonverbal behavior and sensitivity in the context of attachment relationships. *Journal of Nonverbal Behavior*, (29)3, 141–169, 10.1007/s10919-005-4847-x

Schröder, A., Rehfeld, E., ... and Fink, P. (2012). Cognitive-behavioural group treatment for a range of functional somatic syndromes: randomised trial. *British Journal of Psychiatry*, 200, 499–507.

Segal, Z. V., Williams, J. M. G., and Teasdale, J. D. (2002). *Mindfulness-Based Cognitive Therapy for Depression: A New Approach to Preventing Relapse.* Guilford.

Selders, M., Visser, R. ... and Koelen, J. A. (2015). The development of a brief group intervention (Dynamic Interpersonal Therapy) for patients with medically unexplained somatic symptoms: a pilot study, *Psychoanalytic Psychotherapy*, 29(2), 182–198, doi: 10.1080/02668734.2015.1036106

Smith, E., Murphy, J., and Coats, S. (1999). Attachment to groups: theory and management. *Journal of Personality and Social Psychology*, (77) 94–110.

Smith, G. R., Monson, R. A., and Ray, D. C. (1986). Patients with multiple unexplained symptoms: their characteristics, functional health, and health care utilization. *Archives of Internal Medicine*, 146, 69–72.

Sochos, A. (2015). Beyond interpersonal relationships: Attachment to social groups, ideological systems, and social institutions. *The Psychologist*, 28, 986–991.

Spertus, I. L., Yehuda, R., ... and Seremetis, S. V. (2003). Childhood emotional abuse and neglect as predictors of psychological and physical symptoms in women presenting to a primary care practice. *Child Abuse Neglect*, 27, 1247–1258.

Stalker, C. A., and Davies, F. (1995). Attachment organization and adaptation in sexually abused women. *Canadian J. Psychiatry*, 40, 234–240.

Steinbrecher, N., Koerber, S., Frieser, D., and Hiller, W. (2011). The prevalence of medically unexplained symptoms in primary care. *Psychosomatics*, May–Jun; 52(3), 263–271. doi:10.1016/j.psym.2011.01.007.

Stuart, S., and Noyes, R. (1999). Attachment and interpersonal communication in somatization. *Psychosomatics*, 40, 34–43.

Taylor, R. E., Mann, A. H., White, N. J., and Goldberg, D. P. (2000). Attachment style in patients with unexplained physical complaints. *Psychological Medicine*, 30, 931–941.

Taylor, R. E., Marshall, T., Mann, A., and Goldberg, D. P. (2012). Insecure attachment and frequent attendance in primary care: a longitudinal cohort study of medically unexplained symptom presentations in ten UK general practices. *Psychological Medicine*, Apr; 42(4), 855–864. doi: 10.1017/S0033291711001589. Epub 2011 Aug 31.

Tremblay, I., and Sullivan, M. J. L. (2010). Attachment and pain outcome in adolescents: the mediating role of pain catastrophizing and anxiety, *J. Pain*, 11, 160–171.

Van der Kolk, B. (2015). *The Body Keeps the Score: Mind, Brain and Body in the Transformation of Trauma.* Penguin Books.

Van Ravesteijn, H. J., Suijkerbuijk, Y. B., ... and Speckens, A. E. M. (2014). Mindfulness-based cognitive therapy (MBCT) for patients with medically unexplained symptoms: process of change. *Psychosomatic Research*, Jul; 77(1), 27–33. doi: 10.1016/j.jpsychores.2014.04.010. Epub 2014 May 5.

Verhaak, P. F., Meijer, S. A., Visser, A. P., and Wolters, G. (2006). Persistent presentation of medically unexplained symptoms in general practice. *Family Practice*, 23, 414–420. 10.1093/fampra/cml016.

Vesterling, C., and Koglin, U. (2020). The relationship between attachment and somatoform symptoms in children and adolescents: a systematic review and meta-analysis. *Psychosomatic Research*, 130. https://doi.org/10.1016/j.jpsychores.2020.109932

Waldinger, R. J., Schulz, M.S., ... and Ahern, D. K. (2006). Mapping the road from childhood trauma to adult somatization: the role of attachment. *Psychosomatic Medicine*, 68, 129–35.

Waller, E., Scheidt, C. E., and Hartmann, A. (2004). Attachment representation and illness behavior in somatoform disorders. *Journal of Nervous and Mental Disease*, 192, 200–209.

Wallin, D. J. (2017). *Attachment in Psychotherapy*. Guilford Press.

White, K. (2004). *Touch: Attachment and the Body*. Karnac.

Yoshihara, K., Hiramoto, T., ... and Sudo, N. (2014). Effect of 12 weeks of yoga training on the somatization, psychological symptoms, and stress-related biomarkers of healthy women. *Biopsychosocial Medicine*, Jan; 38(1), 1. doi: 10.1186/ 1751-0759-8-1.

Zonneveld, L. N. L., van Rood, Y. R., ... and Busschbach, J. J. V. (2012). Effective group training for patients with unexplained physical symptoms: a randomized controlled trial with a non-randomized one-year follow-up. *PloS ONE*, 012; 7(8): e42629. doi: 10.1371/journal.pone.0042629

Chapter 8

Student Stress, Somatisation and Mental Health

(A version of this chapter was first published by Payne, H. [2022] entitled The BodyMind Approach to Support Students in Higher Education: The Relationship between Student Stress, Somatisation and Mental Health in *Innovations in Education and Teaching International*, 59(4), 483–494)

Introduction

This article proposes that The BodyMind Approach® (TBMA) (Payne, 2009) can be employed as an innovative psychoeducational and biopsychosocial intervention targeting the many students in universities with medically unexplained symptoms (MUS) (such as chronic pain/fatigue, fibromyalgia, headache or backache), often with co-occurring anxiety/depression. It provides a rationale for TBMA by exploring benefits in the context of the relationships between student stress, MUS and the substantial increase in mental ill-health in higher education providers (HEP). By contributing to the discussion on how to enhance student help-seeking behaviour for chronic stress/mental health difficulties, TBMA has the potential to advance knowledge and facilitate theory development in mental health within HEPs. As we have seen earlier in the book, TBMA has shown encouraging outcomes in the UK National Health Service (Payne & Brooks, 2017, 2018, 2020).

There is a cultivation of good mental health and sustained resilience through participants learning to self-manage stress associated with MUS, by integrating body with mind in TBMA. Previous studies on body-oriented approaches for MUS (Röhricht et al., 2019; Papadopoulos et al., 2017) employing dance movement psychotherapy showed positive results. Students may be more able to live well with their bodily distress by learning to self-manage, rather than face consequences such as reduced emotional resilience and/or mental health conditions due to overwhelming stress. TBMA could contribute to overall mental health and wellbeing by, for example, increasing early help-seeking behaviour and academic outcomes. Furthermore, it may reduce referrals to oversubscribed student counselling services and/or withdrawals from studies. It is hoped this discourse will help inform organisational practices and educational policies aimed at supporting student mental health and wellbeing.

DOI: 10.4324/9781003460749-9

The BodyMind Approach in the Context of Higher Education and Student Mental Health

Current HEPs' wellbeing interventions address solely the psychological elements of MUS. This, despite almost half of students feeling unable to access such services due to stigma, defensive verbal communication to avoid emotion, their explanatory model of chronic bodily symptoms being solely physical or their being non-native speakers. Medication/pain management treats these bodily symptoms but neglects the associated stress/anxiety/depression. No current intervention caters for *both* the emotional and bodily distress, attracts less stigma, reduces avoidance behaviour or employs nonverbal, embodied methods as opposed to verbal language alone. Since many students do not disclose/ seek help for chronic stress/mental health difficulties, a psychoeducational intervention targeting students with MUS may be more acceptable, reducing fear of judgement and thus increasing numbers benefiting from support.

The BodyMind Approach is designed for students not coping with their MUS to learn to self-manage both symptoms, and the emotional counterpart, to improve and sustain good mental health. The conceptual framework proposed highlights how an innovative, holistic TBMA learning and teaching programme, addressing the inter-relationship of body with mind, might contribute to an integrated, whole-university approach towards student mental health.

Figure 8.1 below is a suggested whole university model with a central referral hub to triage student needs for support. It integrates mental health and wellbeing with specialisms such as the academic and personal tutor.

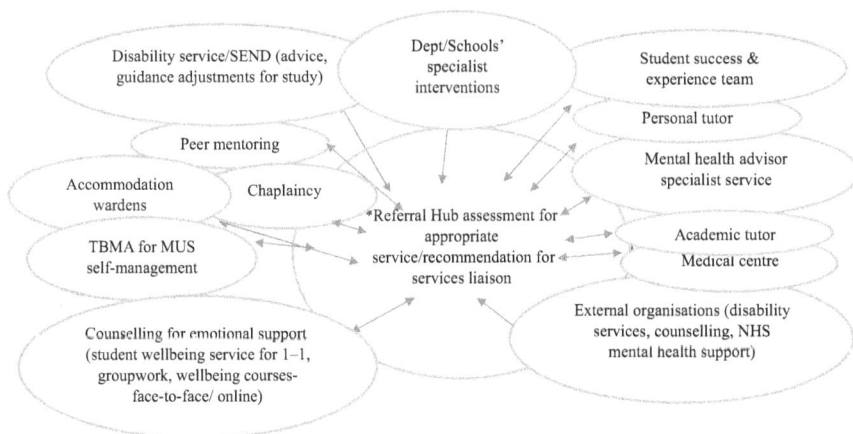

Figure 8.1   Plugging the gap in support for students with MUS in an integrated mental health and wellbeing strategy

*Individual services signpost students to the referral/triaging hub. Following an assessment, the hub refers to an appropriate service and, if appropriate, recommends liaison between services.

With reference to TBMA specifically, classes comprise 12 two-hourly sessions over ten weeks. The first two weeks are held twice per week (as outlined in Chapter 4). Pre- and post-monitoring, and formulation of a tailor-made action plan for the embedment of self-management strategies over the subsequent six months are included. From piloting TBMA training online, delivery of TBMA online for students is possible.

The model employs embodied, enactive practices such as bodymindfulness, movement, writing, mark-making or collage to help make meaning from sensory experiencing in the body. By exploring symptoms, and associated emotions, and practising tracking these, "signals", sent by the body about emotions, the relationship with symptoms can change. For example, learning to notice subtle tightening or retreating in the body is a response to a possible threatening situation (Craig, 2002; Dael, Mortillaro & Scherer, 2012). Becoming conscious of, and receptive to, this interoceptive response can lead to feelings of control, agency and emotional resilience. TBMA promotes kind attention to bodily sensations, monitoring signals from interoceptive awareness, with an exploratory interest, rather than emotional reactivity and negative appraisal. Attention towards interaction between sensation, emotions, images and thoughts, supports body with mind connectivity. Movement is an innate mechanism for auto/self-regulation (Shafir, 2015). An increased awareness of movement can support emotional regulation towards internal/external stimuli, giving more choice and skills to adapt, so needs are met.

This model appears acceptable and more accessible to people experiencing MUS than psychological/talking therapy (Payne & Brooks, 2020). Research (N=90) shows TBMA can sustain engagement (97%); reliably reduce symptom distress (63%), anxiety (42%) and depression (35%); and increase overall activity (58%), wellbeing (55%) and functioning (35%) (Payne & Stott, 2010; Payne, 2014), sustained over six months (Payne and Brooks, 2017).

Approaches that integrate practices to promote multiple dimensions of students' wellbeing, such as the bidirectionality of body with mind, are limited (Moses, Bradley & O'Callaghan, 2016). Stress reduction, counselling and mindfulness therapies focus on reducing anxiety/depression (Church, De Asis &Brooks, 2012; Deckro, Ballinger &Benson, 2002; Regehr, Glancy & Pitts, 2013). However, they ignore chronic symptoms and are usually conducted individually, whereas group support focusing on both symptom- and emotional-distress, found in TBMA, helps reverse isolation. Interventions targeting pain, self-help/social support, wellbeing, academic performance, resilience, persistence and retention ignore psychological aspects (Mattanah et al., 2012; Robbins et al., 2009). TBMA addresses both physical and emotional health simultaneously by firstly working with the bodily distress, which subsequently leads to behavioural change, i.e. self-management of the symptom (dis)stress-response.

Endorsed as a class or workshop for learning to manage symptoms, TBMA may seem more appealing to students than counselling/psychological approaches. Promoted as supporting sustained wellbeing in body and mind, helping the learning process, improving grades and preventing excessive stress, TBMA may increase help-seeking behaviour. TBMA classes might prevent any associated mental health difficulties from escalating, or even occurring since MUS may be a precursor for anxiety and/or depression. There is likely a dynamic between mental health and MUS.

The advantages of TBMA include reducing a) the possibility of new conditions, b) exacerbation of existing concerns, c) isolation d) anxiety/depression, e) symptom distress and f) GP/hospital visits. Furthermore, TBMA may increase a) activity, b) wellbeing, and c) feelings of control when living with uncertainty (Payne & Brooks, 2017; Payne, Jarvis & Roberts, 2019).

Stress and Its Relationship to Student Mental Health

Whilst stress is part of life, people respond, and experience it, differently. Any threat towards something cared about, such as employment, results in stress. Threats or stress are due to demands exceeding the capacity to cope. The initial stress reaction is helpful – alerting us to what matters, allowing us to find our comfort-zone or change our lives to cope. When stressors are excessive, multiple and sustained, they can reduce mental health and cause bodily symptoms (Clarke, 2016). Vulnerability to excessive stress can result in poor emotional self-regulation, reduced resilience to manage, and/or MUS/mental health difficulties (for example, depression/ generalised anxiety).

A history of trauma can lead to a pre-disposition for stress overflowing. When potential threats are perceived, such as students feeling out of control due to academic demands, transition, uncertainty or isolation, the stress response kicks-in. When that threat feels bigger than the capacity to cope, the stress response gets stuck in the body. The unconscious body-brain wants to avoid that situation repeating, so, if a similar situation/or felt-experience to past trauma is involved, the reptilian brain responds in that same way.

Targeting vulnerable student groups may help to prevent high stress levels avoiding mental ill-health (Universities UK, 2019) and/or MUS (Kroenke & Price, 1993). TBMA, by supporting students to learn to manage stress through managing their MUS (via self/body compassion), and emotional regulation, may improve students' resilience and ability to cope with threats (De la Fuente, Fernández-Cabezas & Mattila, 2008). Some new factors involved in these higher student stress levels leading to increased mental health concerns, and/or MUS, are presented as a context and rationale for delivering TBMA in HEPs.

New Factors Affecting Student Stress Levels

Students have always experienced stress, but in the UK nowadays there is more due to new, complex and multi-faceted factors, leading to, or exacerbating, mental health conditions or impacting students vulnerable to stress.

The rise in the percentage of children and young people with mental health difficulties in England, and worldwide (McGorry et al., 2024), together with the widening participation government policy for HEPs, has resulted in more students entering with a diagnosis, or with fragile mental health. Consequently, any increase in stressors may have a knock-on effect on already delicate mental health.

The government's policy of 50% of all young people entering HEPs led to growing numbers of students from disadvantaged backgrounds. This policy is measured by the Higher Education Statistics Authority/HESA (2018) using indicators of: a) low neighbourhood HEP participation, b) parents not having attended HEPs and c) increased enrolment from state schools/colleges. Poor mental health in disadvantaged populations (social, economic, cultural or political) is higher (Meyer, Schwartz & Frost, 2008) and associated with substantially greater risks of common mental health conditions (House of Commons Education, Health & Social Care Committee, 2018), and MUS (Kroenke & Price, 1993). These students experience more stressors, such as likely feeling more isolated, increased pressure to succeed, less support and poorer financial security (Williams, Coare & Anderson, 2015; Bennett et al., 2023). This exposes them to stress overflowing, resulting in mental ill-health and/or MUS. Indeed, reports from this policy anticipated increased mental health difficulties (Department for Business, Innovation & Skills, 2013).

Early research suggests change and transition are stressful (Hobfoll & Walfisch, 1986). Students have always had to adjust to substantial change transitioning to unfamiliar HEPs when growing from adolescence to adulthood, dependence to independence, acclimatising to changes in lifestyle and increased study demands. Since greater numbers now are fragile to mental health difficulties, change/transitions can be more problematic. Leaving supportive family, friends, school, usually going to a strange city with unknown people – these can tip the balance for students who previously managed. When transitioning to HEPs, returning from vacation or going on placement, stress will be experienced positively or negatively depending on mental health history.

Economic factors can be a stressor, for example, where a full-time student is having to work due to lack of parental financial contribution to the maintenance loan. The rise in tuition fees (covered by a student loan viewed as a debt) results in partial increases in undergraduates' mental health difficulties (Richardson, Elliott & Roberts, 2015). Debt links to poorer psychological functioning and students considering withdrawing (Cooke et al., 2004; Walsemann, Gee & Gentile, 2015).

The competitive employment market pressurises students to gain the highest degree level. An increase of only 10% of graduate jobs has occurred since 2001, and, in the third quarter of 2017 49% of all recent graduates worked in non-graduate roles (Office for National Statistics/ONS, 2017). This shortfall will likely increase substantially in the forthcoming years.

Any combination of these factors can be additional stressors contributing to increased student mental ill-health. This is especially hard to cope with if feeling unsupported, already fragile to excessive stress, and experiencing a diagnosed/undiagnosed mental health concern and/or MUS. TBMA, in supporting students to self-manage MUS, may not only decrease excessive stress, but sustain robust, emotional health and wellbeing and increase connection with the collective.

Interoception and Stress/Anxiety

Multiple psychological and biomedical theories have been proposed to explain MUS. They highlight dysfunctional stress responses across various physiological axes (such as the hypothalamic-pituitary-adrenal axis, inflammatory responses, and cardiovascular responses). Additionally, interoceptive dysregulation is highlighted although knowledge of these interactions is still inadequate. The research often focuses on a single mechanism, stress test, physiological stress axis or specific MUS condition. This leads to fragmented understanding whereas MUS may have a similar underlying aetiology.

Interoception (the experience of feeling sensations inside the body) has been recognised to play a role in mental health. A primary dysfunction in perception and regulation of bodily states has been considered in emotional processing (Seth & Friston, 2016; Petzschner et al. 2021,) e.g., anxiety (Paulus & Stein 2010; Herbert & Pollatos, 2012; Stephan et al., 2016). In a review by Khalsa et al. (2018) findings show a lack of interoception adversely affects mood disorders, addictions, and post-traumatic stress disorder (PTSD), among many other mental health issues. Others argue that the interoceptive predictions are resistant to update self-models and this results in an un-ease of self in the world or given contexts which is experienced as anxiety/distress (Nord & Garfinkel, 2022; Sugawara et al., 2020). Whilst we do not know whether interoception will provide the necessary mechanism to reduce anxiety/overwhelming stress, PTSD is a form of anxiety/fear response to the threat of survival. This is suggestive of potential for an intervention focusing on interoception for reducing anxiety/overwhelming stress. What is known is that interoceptive awareness can mediate the relationship between stress and emotion according to Craig (2002) and between anxiety and the intensity of unpleasant feelings (Pollatos et al., 2007).

Interoception may occur below the level of consciousness albeit extending beyond immediate physiological responses (Durán, Morales & Huepe, 2024). It is interconnected with impulsive processes, affective states, motivations, adaptive reactions, cognition and emotional experiences, all of which play pivotal roles in maintaining homeostatic balance, regulating bodily functions and ensuring survival (Khalsa et al., 2018). When homeostasis is out of balance, signals from the body reach the level of consciousness (e.g., when breathing or heart rate increase due to panic attacks, anxiety and stress) (Berntson and Khalsa, 2021).

Based on findings from computational neuroscience and active inference approaches (Friston, Daunizeau & Kiebel et al., 2009), the somatic error hypothesis of anxiety (Khalsa & Feinstein, 2018) states that anxiety-related distress arises due to the discrepancy between the actual and anticipated, but habitually based, bodily state. Via feedforward and feedback loops, interoceptive perceptions are dynamically and interactively co-created by the body and the brain. Importantly, the actual incoming sensations from the ascending afferent pathways (bottom-up signalling) can be altered by the brain's anticipated sensation (top-down signalling). This is based on prior experiences. Individuals who experience chronic anxiety-related distress seem to have lost the ability to accurately sense what is happening in the body. This contributes to an increasing sense of dysregulation and threat even in the absence of such (Paulus, Feinstein & Khalsa, 2019; Nord & Garfinkel, 2022). Thus, interventions that target interoceptive mechanisms may be pivotal for efficacious treatment. Recent research reveals efficacy for reducing anxiety via interoceptive training (Garfinkel, Mclanachan & Crtichley, 2017; Sugawara et al., 2020; Harrison et al., 2021).

The BodyMind Approach works with the felt sense experience of movement from bodily signals/sensation through interoception practices to reduce and integrate the stress response. By practising tracking this moving experience in the body, any "somatic markers/signals" (Damasio, 2000) sent by the body about emotions can be more readily perceived. This raises both emotional and body awareness. Becoming conscious of, and receptive to, this response can lead to agency (feelings of control) and emotional resilience by strengthening the perception of the actual body state. This thereby reduces somatic errors which underlie anxious symptomatology. For example, hypervigilance toward disturbed body states, abnormal self-related thinking patterns and attempts to reduce these aversive experiences via avoidance or escape behaviours (Khalsa & Feinstein, 2018). Movement is an innate mechanism for self-regulation (Shafir, 2015). An increased awareness of bodily movement can support responses to internal/external stimuli, giving more choice and skills to adapt so needs are met. Participants make meaning from sensory experiencing in the body to feel more in control and to self-manage. The programme for TBMA is multi-model, involving creative, active and bodymindfulness practices, progressive relaxation, expressive movement, writing, mark-making on paper as a form of reflection and languaging of the experience.

Specifically, TBMA supports:

- a more accurate interpretation of the somatic signals;
- the identification and exploration of somatic markers often emerging from the stress-response to threat;

- self-management through cultivating connection between the body and the mind;
- making meaning from the sensory experience through aesthetic practices to provide much needed understanding leading to a sense of control;
- practising of protective strategies to inform behaviour change; and
- preventing the escalation of anxiety/overwhelming stress into a chronic mental health condition.

Student Stress and Medically Unexplained Symptoms

Just as MUS can lead to, and is associated with, excessive stress (Mobini, 2015), high stress levels can result in MUS, and mental and/or physical illnesses (Schneiderman, Ironson & Siegel, 2005). In a University College London (UCL) Union survey students complained of anxiety, depression, physical pain and insomnia, in that order (UCL, 2019). If students complain of the physical symptoms of excessive stress almost as much as the emotional ones, then TBMA can effectively support both. Physical symptoms (for example, pain, insomnia, eye twitching, fatigue) alert us to the effects of a threat/pressure, i.e. a stress response in the body. TBMA can educate students to notice and understand these signals to learn how to self-manage stress, hopefully before symptoms (another stress) overflow to trigger mental health difficulties and/or develop into chronic MUS.

One in six GP consultations are for MUS (Rosendal et al., 2015; Steinbrecher et al., 2011). MUS mostly affects women, young people (Steinbrecher et al., 2011; Nimnuan, Hotopf & Wessely, 2001; Reid et al., 2002) and non-native speakers (Verhaak et al., 2006), all of which number highly in the student population. There is a high prevalence of MUS in students, often with co-occurring anxiety, depression and chronic stress (Henningsen, Zimmermann & Sattel, 2003). Consequently, MUS it is an important area of concern related to improving student mental health/wellbeing.

Treatment for MUS is normally via mental health services but for only the most severe presentations of IBS with anxiety/depression (Laird et al., 2016). Alternatively, there is graded exercise for chronic fatigue (Cochrane Database of Systematic Review, 2008). Most MUS sufferers find mental health routes unacceptable due to their explanatory model as physical, rather than psychological (Heijmans, Olde Hartman & van Weel, 2011). The BodyMind Approach focuses on the stress-experience of the symptoms; firstly, it is attractive to participants, fitting with this mind-set. We can assume students are no different in this case.

When adaptive stress responses kick-in, previous unresolved threats to survival, safety or wellbeing are stimulated, and unwanted stress pours into the "stress bucket". The result can be a chronic stress state, often manifesting as MUS, causing even more stress (as the threat is in the body) in a downward spiral if interruption to the iterative cycle is unforthcoming (Mobini, 2015).

The BodyMind Approach is designed to interfere with this cycle, realigning body with mind for healthier functioning, and overall wellbeing. Symptom distress can be the tipping point for future deterioration and complex mental health conditions if not addressed early (Chew-Graham, Heyland & Sumathipala, 2017). Yet, so far, there is no early pathway for learning self-management of MUS in HEPs. The BodyMind Approach can fill this gap. In the context of student mental health, an understanding of the ramifications of excessive stress in student life is important when considering how to address this critical issue. Excessive stress, MUS and mental health are inextricably related. To stem the substantial rise in student mental health concerns, undue stress and associated MUS, HEPs need appropriate interventions.

Student Mental Health

Student mental health difficulties have grown immensely, mirroring the rise in the diagnosis of children and young people (NHS Digital, 2018). From 2,169 applicants, and 6,504 current students, 12% reported mental health difficulties, 32% "often/always" felt down/depressed in the previous four weeks, and 30% "often/always" felt isolated/lonely (Unite, 2016). Over the last ten years the number of student suicides has risen (ONS, 2018), and attrition rates grown due to mental ill-health (Marsh, 2017). One in four students reported mental health problems (YouGov, 2016), and nearly five times as many as ten years ago disclosed a mental health condition (Thorley, 2017). Since the COVID-19 pandemic these numbers have increased even more.

Mental health difficulties peak between 16–24 years, overlapping the median age of students. Kessler, Berglund & Walters (2005) found 64% of students (and 83% of undergraduates) are between 16–24 years, as today, with 75% of mental health problems established by age 25. The increased numbers in this age range results in more mental health difficulties, driven by women who are almost three times more likely to experience mental ill-health than men. The proportion of 16–24-year-old women students with mental health difficulties increased by 38% from 1993–2014, whereas it decreased by 3% for 16–24-year-old men (NHS Digital, 2014). Since 2015, more women than men have consistently entered UK universities (Higher Education Statistics Agency/HESA, 2018). Consequently, with widening participation, more women than men are entering HEPs with a diagnosed/undiagnosed mental health condition. Mostly women participated in TBMA health-service deliveries so TBMA could contribute to improving the mental health/MUS conditions of women students.

In England students have worse mental health outcomes compared to their non-student peers, particularly in marginalised communities (McCloud et al., 2023). Recent events, such as the COVID-19 pandemic, have taken a further toll on mental health (Frampton & Smithies, 2021). Yet the data indicates a growing number of students reporting mental health difficulties which is the main reason students withdraw from their studies (approximately 25% more frequently than any other reason (Sanders, 2023).

In the last decade, students disclosing a mental health condition to their university increased sevenfold (Lewis & Bolton, 2023), also reflected in the Universities and Colleges Admissions Service (UCAS) where there was a 45% rise in applicants reporting a mental health concern since 2011 (UCAS, 2021). A UK survey of over 12,000 students from 147 universities found four in five students experienced mental health difficulties, an increase from three in five since 2021 (Marris et al., 2022). Another found 57% reported having a current mental health concern. However, not all students reported this to their university, with one in four not knowing where to go to get mental health support at university if they needed it (Student Minds, 2023). It should be noted universities have been successfully sued for psychological damages after failing to accommodate mental health (Petkar, 2017; Weale, 2023).

The increase in student mental ill-health is not solely in the UK. In the USA, Soet and Sevig (2006) explored the history, coping and mental health distress levels in one university, and provided recommendations for research, policy and practice. Kitzrow (2009) acknowledged the needs and challenges posed by the increase in students with serious psychological problems seeking counselling onsite. Iarovici (2014) raised concerns that student mental health was becoming a crisis for HEPs.

The UK media highlighted the increase in undergraduate mental health difficulties (Marsh, 2017), although students have always had mental health difficulties. As far back as Roberts et al. (1999), student mental health in two London universities was substantially lower than in the general population, supported later by Stallman (2010). Cooke et al. (2006) found mental health levels never returned to those of pre-enrolment in 4,699 students. Webb et al. (1996) reported student anxiety at 54%, and depression at 13%; and Bewick et al. (2008) also found anxiety higher than depression for 1,129 students. Andrews and Wilding (2004) surveyed 351 students one month before starting university and at mid-course. Nine percent of those with no symptoms before university had depression, and 20% had clinically significant anxiety by mid-course. In a year, a quarter of students reported psychological distress associated with increased risk of anxiety, depression, substance abuse and personality disorders (Verger et al., 2009). Anxiety, associated with excessive stress, appears to be a major concern for students.

Only 27% of students thought their university provided adequate mental health support (NatWest Student Living Index, 2020). The Equality Challenge Unit (2014) found half experiencing mental health difficulties had not received support. Furthermore, almost half with difficulties were unwilling to disclose/ seek treatment, fearing other students thinking less of them or of receiving unfair treatment from their institution. The biggest challenges for students with mental health difficulties seeking help were fearing judgements and being shown as weak (Byrom, 2014). TBMA circumnavigates these barriers since it engages students based on their MUS, rather than their mental health/stress presentation. There is safety in self-referring to an intervention for overtly presenting physical symptoms, rather than for mental health, and when the programme is perceived as a class for learning, rather than as psychological therapy for mental health concerns. The fears evaporate, so participants can sustain involvement over 12 sessions.

Summary

Mental health difficulties will continue to increase for students (NHS Digital, 2018). Higher education policies and wellbeing services have a long way to go in their legal duty of care to avoid harm, provide support and co-produce strategies to support mental health. There is an opportunity now to consider joined up approaches to transform cultures and embed initiatives beyond wellbeing services. This may improve help-seeking, decrease isolation and promote a shared purpose for good mental health. Leaving students to struggle may result in more mental health difficulties, increased distress for those already diagnosed and the onset of more chronic, debilitating MUS.

Stones and Glazzard (2019) recommend an institution-wide approach to eradicate stigma, enabling students to be mentally healthy, and extending beyond provisions targeting solely mental ill-health. TBMA fits into this extended provision. There are overlaps between the body, mind and aspects of wellbeing (Checkoway, 2011). These overlaps could be captured by TBMA at times of increased stress such as induction, before/after transitions, placements, examinations and deadlines. TBMA may reduce stigma and attend to students' physical (and emotional) distress as part of an overall mental health and wellbeing strategy based in student services/faculties/schools. It will be crucial to research TBMA in this new context of HEP, as well as its outcomes, the referral system and the student population, as all differ from TBMA delivery in the health service.

There are unique opportunities now with the UK University Mental Health Charter (Hughes and Spanner, 2019) and Student Mental Health Manifesto (Student Minds, 2024) to review the way student mental health is regarded, and which evidence-based interventions are accessible and acceptable to *all* students, not only those able to engage with student wellbeing services. The Office for Students (OfS) allocated funding to support the rising demand for the University Mental Health Charter, emphasising the government's commitment to improving student mental health across HEPs (Department of Education, 2018; OfS, 2024).

References

Andrews, B., and Wilding, J., M. (2004). The relation of depression and anxiety to life-stress and achievement in students. *British Journal of Psychology*, 95 (Pt4), 509–521. doi: 10.1348/0007126042369802

Bennett, J., Heron, J., Kidger, J and Myles-Jay, L. (2023) Investigating change in student financial stress at a UK university: multi-year survey analysis across a global pandemic and recession. *Education Sciences*, 13, 1175. https://doi.org/10.3390/educsci13121175

Berntson, G. G., and Khalsa, S. S. (2021). Neural circuits of interoception. *Trends Neurosci.* 44, 17–28. doi: 10.1016/j.tins.2020.09.011

Bewick, B. M., Gill, J. and Mulhern, B. (2008) Using electronic surveying to assess psychological distress within the UK university student population: a multi-site pilot investigation. *E-Journal of Applied Psychology*, 4(2), 1–5. https://doi.org/10.7790/ejap.v4i2.120

Byrom, N. (2014). Grand challenges in student mental health report. Student Minds. http://www.studentminds.org.uk/uploads/3/7/8/4/3784584/grand_challenges_report_for_public.pdf

Checkoway, B. (2011). New perspectives on civic engagement and psychosocial well-being. *Liberal Education*, 97(2), 6–11.

Chew-Graham, C. A., Heyland, S., and Sumathipala, A. (2017) Medically unexplained symptoms: Continuing challenges for primary care. *British Journal of General Practice*, 67(656), 106–107. doi.org/10.3399/bjgp17X689473

Church, D., De Asis, M. A., and Brooks, A. J. (2012). Brief group intervention using Emotional Freedom Techniques for depression in college students: A randomized controlled trial. *Depression Research and Treatment*, vol. 2012, Article ID 257172, 1–7. doi:10.1155/2012/257172. https://www.hindawi.com/journals/drt/2012/257172/

Clarke, D. D. (2016). Solving medical mysteries: Hidden stresses and unexplained symptoms. *Slovenian J. of Public Health* (Zdr Varst), Sep 1; 55(3), 152–154. doi: 10.1515/sjph-2016-0029.

Cochrane Database of Systematic Reviews. (2008). *Cognitive Behaviour Therapy for Chronic Fatigue Syndrome*. First published: July 16 by Cochrane Publications.

Cooke, R., Barkham, B. M., … and Davy, J. (2004) Student debt and its relation to student mental health. *J. Further and Higher Education*, 28, 1, 53–66. doi: 10.1080/0309877032000161814

Cooke, R., Bewick, B. M., … and Audin, K. (2006) Measuring, monitoring and managing the psychological well-being of first year university students. *British J. Guidance and Counselling*, 34, 4, 505–517. doi: 10.1080/03069880600942624.

Craig, A. D. (2002). How do you feel? Interoception: the sense of the physiological condition of the body. *National Review Neuroscience*, 3,, 655–666. doi: 10.1038/nrn894.

Dael, N., Mortillaro, M., and Scherer, K. R. (2012). Emotion expression in body action and posture. *Emotion* 12, 5, 1085–1101. doi: 10.1037/a0025737.

Damasio, A. (2000). *The Feeling of What Happens: Body, Emotion and the Making of Consciousness*. Vintage.

De la Fuente, J., Fernández-Cabezas, M., and Mattila, P. (2008). Evaluations of an organisational stress management program in a municipal public works' organisations. *Occupational Health Psychology*, 13(1), 10–23.

Deckro, G. R., Ballinger, K. M., and Benson, H. (2002). The evaluation of a mind/body intervention to reduce psychological distress and perceived stress in college students. *American College Health*, 50(6), 281–287. doi:10.1080/07448480209603446

Department for Business Innovation and Skills. (2013). *Widening Participation in Higher Education.* https://www.gov.uk/government/collections/widening-participation-in-higher-education

Department for Education. (2018). *New Package of Measures Announced on Student Mental Health.* https://www.gov.uk/government/news/new-package-of-measures-announced-on-student-mental-health

Durán, S. P., Morales J.-P. and Huepe, D. (2024). Interoceptive awareness in a clinical setting: the need to bring interoceptive perspectives into clinical evaluation.*ront. Psychol.* 15:1244701. doi: 10.3389/fpsyg.2024.1244701

Equality Challenge Unit. (2014). *Understanding Adjustments: Supporting Staff and Students Who Are Experiencing Mental Health Difficulties.* https://www.ecu.ac.uk/publications/understanding-adjustments-mental-health/

Frampton, N., and Smithies, D. (2021). University Mental Health: Life in a Pandemic. Student Minds. https://www.studentminds.org.uk/uploads/3/7/8/4/3784584/2021_ir_full_report_final.pdf

Friston K. J., Daunizeau, J. and Kiebel, S. (2009) Reinforcement learning or active inference? *PLoS ONE,* 4, e6421.

Garfinkel, S., Mclanachan, A. and Critchley, H. D. (2017). Interoceptive training for anxiety management in autism: aligning dimension of interoceptive experience, ADIE (c). *Psychosom,* 79(4).

Harrison, O. K. ... and Stephan, K. E. (2021). Interoception of breathing and its relationship with anxiety. *Neuron.* 15; 109(24), 4080–4093.e8.

Heijmans, M., Olde Hartman, T. C., and van Weel, C. (2011). Experts' opinions on the management of medically unexplained symptoms in primary care. A qualitative analysis of narrative reviews and scientific editorials. *Family Practice,* 28, 4, 444–455.

Henningsen, P., Zimmermann, T., and Sattel, H. (2003). Medically unexplained physical symptoms, anxiety, and depression: A meta-analytic review. *Psychosomatic Medicine,* 65(4), 528–533.

Herbert, B. M. and Pollatos, O. (2012). The body in the mind: on the relationship between interoception and embodiment. *Top. Cogn. Sci.,* 4(4), 692–704.

Higher Education Statistics Agency (HESA). (2018). *Table 15 – UK Domiciled Student Enrolments by Disability and Sex 2016/17* https://www.hesa.ac.uk/data-and-analysis/students/table-15

Hobfoll, S. E., and Walfisch, S. (1986). Stressful event, mastery and depression: a review of crisis theory. *Community Psychology,* 14(2), 183–195.

House of Commons Education Committee and Health and Social Care Committee. (2018). *The Government's Green Paper on Mental Health: Failing a Generation* https://publications.parliament.uk/pa/cm201719/cmselect/cmhealth/642/64207.htm

Hughes, G., and Spanner, L. (2019). *The University Mental Health Charter.* Student Minds.

Iarovici, D. (2014). *Mental Health Issues and the University Student.* Johns Hopkins University Press.

Kessler, R. C., Berglund, P., and Walters, E. E. (2005). Lifetime prevalence and age-of-onset distributions of DSM-IV disorders in the National Comorbidity Survey Replication. *Archives of General Psychiatry,* 62(6), 593–602.

Khalsa S. S., Feinstein S. J. (2018). The somatic error hypothesis of anxiety. In M. Tsakiris and H. De Preester (Eds), *The Interoceptive Mind* (pp. 144–164). Oxford University Press.

Khalsa, S. S. ... and Paulus, M. P. (2018). Interoception and mental health: A roadmap. *Biol. Psych. Cog. Neurosc. and Neuroimaging*, 3(6), 501–513.

Kitzrow, M. A. (2009). The mental health needs of today's college students: Challenges and recommendations. *NASP*, 46(4), 646–660, doi:10.2202/1949-6605.5037

Kroenke, K., and Price, P. K. (1993). Symptoms in the community. *Archives of International Medicine*, 153, 2474–2480. http://dx.doi.org/10.1001/archi nte.1993.00410210102011

Laird, K. T., Tanner-Smith, E. E., ... and Walker, L. S. (2016). Short-term and long-term efficacy of psychological therapies for irritable bowel syndrome: a systematic review and meta-analysis. *Clinical Gastroenterol Hepatol*, 14(7), 937–947.

Lewis, J., and Bolton, P. (2023). Student mental health in England: Statistics, policy, and guidance. UK Parliament. https://commonslibrary.parliament.uk/research-briefings/cbp-8593/

Marris, L., Johnson, R., ... and Hanlon, M. (2022). Student Mental Health Study 2022. *Cibyl*.

Marsh, S. (2017). *Number of University Dropouts Due to Mental Health Problems Trebles* https://www.theguardian.com/society/2017/may/23/number-university-dropouts-due-to-mental-health-problems-trebles#img-1

Mattanah, J. F., Brooks, L. J., ... and Ayers, J. F. (2012). A social support intervention and academic achievement in college: does perceived loneliness mediate the relationship? *College Counseling*, 15(1), 22–36. https://doi:10.1002/jocc.2012.15. issue-1

McCloud, T., Kamenov, S., ... and Lewis, G. (2023). The association between higher education attendance and common mental health problems among young people in England: evidence from two population-based cohorts. *The Lancet Public Health*, 8(10), e811–e819. https://doi.org/10.1016/S2468-2667(23)00188-3

McGorry, D. P., ... and Killackey, E. (2024). The Lancet Psychiatry Commission on youth mental health. *Lancet Psychiatry*, 11, 731–774.

Meyer, I. H., Schwartz, S., and Frost, D. M. (2008) Social patterning of stress and coping: Does disadvantaged social status confer more stress and fewer coping resources? *Social Science Medicine*, 67, 3, 368–79. doi: 10.1016/j.socscimed.2008.03.012

Mobini, S. (2015). Psychology of medically unexplained symptoms: A practical review. *Cogent Psychology*, 2, 1, 1033876 http://dx.doi.org/10.1080/23311 908.2015.1033876

Moses, J., Bradley, G. L., and O'Callaghan, F. V. (2016). When college students look after themselves: self-care practices and well-being. *Student Affairs Research and Practice*, 53(3), 345–359. https://doi:10.1080/19496591.2016.1157488

NatWest. (2020). *NatWest Student Living Index 2020*. https://personal.natwest.com/personal/life-moments/students-and-graduates/student-living-index.html

NHS Digital. (2014). *Adult Psychiatric Morbidity Survey*. https://files.digital.nhs.uk/pdf/q/3/mental_health_and_wellbeing_in_england_full_report.pdf

NHS Digital. (2018). *Mental Health of Children and Young People in England, 2017 [PAS]*. https://digital.nhs.uk/data-and-information/publications/statistical/mental-health-of-children-and-young-people-in-england/2017/2017

Nimnuan, C., Hotopf, M., and Wessely, S. (2001). Medically unexplained symptoms. An epidemiological study in seven specialities, *Psychosomatic Research*, 51, 1, 361–367. doi: 10.1016/s0022-3999(01)00223-9.

Nord, C. L. and Garfinkel, S. N. (2022). Interoceptive pathways to understand and treat mental health conditions. *Trends. Cogn. Sci.* 26(6), 499–513.

Office for Students (OfS). (2024). Funding boost to support Student Minds' University Mental Health Charter. https://www.officeforstudents.org.uk/news-blog-and-eve nts/press-and-media/funding-boost-to-support-student-minds-university-mental-health-charter/

Office of National Statistics. (2017). *Graduates in the UK Labour Market.* https:// www.gov.uk/government/statistics/graduates-in-the-uk-labour-market-2017

Office of National Statistics. (2018). *Estimating Suicide Among Higher Education Students, England and Wales.* https://www.ons.gov.uk/releases/estimatingsuicidea-monghighereducationstudentsenglandandwales

Papadopoulos, N., Burrell, C., Smith, L. and Röhricht, F. (2017). Therapeutic processes and personalised care in body-oriented psychological therapy for patients with medically unexplained symptoms (MUS). *European J. Person Centered Healthcare*, 5(4), 449–453.

Paulus, M. P., Feinstein, J. S., and Khalsa, S. S. (2019). An active inference approach to interoceptive psychopathology. *Annual Review of Clinical Psychology*, 15, 97–122. https://doi.org/10.1146/annurev-clinpsy-050718-095617

Paulus, M. P. and Stein M. B. (2010). Interoception in anxiety and depression. *Brain Struct. Funct.*, 214, 451–463.

Payne, H. (2009). Pilot study to evaluate dance movement psychotherapy (the BodyMind Approach) with patients with medically unexplained symptoms: participant and facilitator perceptions and a summary discussion. *Body, Movement and Dance in Psychotherapy*, 5(2), 95–106.

Payne, H. (2014). Patient experience: push past symptom mysteries. *The Health Service Journal*, 124(6390), 26–27.

Payne, H., and Brooks, S. (2017). Moving on: The BodyMind Approach™ for medically unexplained symptoms (outcomes). *Public Mental Health*, 16, 2. doi: 10.1108/ JPMH-10-2016-0052

Payne, H., and Brooks, S. (2018). Different strokes for different folks: The BodyMind Approach as a learning tool for patients with medically unexplained symptoms to self-manage. *Frontiers in Psychology.* https://doi.org/10.3389/ fpsyg.2018.02222

Payne, H., and Brooks, S. (2020). A qualitative study of the views of patients with medically unexplained symptoms on The BodyMind Approach®: employing embodied methods and arts practices for self-management. *Frontiers in Psychology.* https:// doi.org/10.3389/fpsyg.2020.554566

Payne, H., Jarvis, J., and Roberts, A. (2019). The BodyMind Approach® as transformative learning to promote self-management for patients with medically unexplained symptoms. *Transformative Education*, 18, 2, 114–147. https://doi.org/ 10.1177/1541344619883892

Payne, H., and Stott, D. (2010). Change in the moving bodymind: Quantitative results from a Pilot study on the BodyMind Approach (BMA) as groupwork for patients with medically unexplained symptoms (MUS). *Counselling and Psychotherapy Research*, 10(4), 295–307. https://doi.org/10.1080/14733140903551645

Petkar, S. (2017) Students sue Oxford University amid claims of mental health discrimination. *The Express*, August 8. https://www.express.co.uk/news/uk/838522/mental-health-oxford-university-discrimination-students-sue-jesus-college

Petzschner, F. H. ... and Khalsa, S. S. (2021). Computational models of interoception and body regulation. *Trends Neurosci.*, 44, 63–76.

Pollatos, O. et al., (2007). Interoceptive awareness mediates the relationship between anxiety and the intensity of unpleasant feelings. *J. Anxiety Disord.*, 21(7): 931–43.

Regehr, C., Glancy, D., and Pitts, A. (2013). Interventions to reduce stress in university students: A review and meta-analysis. *Affective Disorders*, 148(1), 1–11. https://doi:10.1016/j.jad.2012.11.026

Reid, S., Wessely, S., Crayford, T., and Hotopf, M. (2002). Frequent attenders with medically unexplained symptoms: service use and costs in secondary care. *British J. Psychiatry*, 180, 248–253. doi: 10.1192/bjp.180.3.248

Richardson, T., Elliott, P., and Roberts, R. (2015). The impact of tuition fees' amount on mental health over time in British students. *Public Health*, 37(3), 1, 412–418, https://doi.org/10.1093/pubmed/fdv003

Robbins, S. B., Oh, I., Le, H., and Button, C. (2009). Intervention effects on college performance and retention as mediated by motivational, emotional, and social control factors: Integrated meta-analytic path analyses. *Applied Psychology*, 94(5), 1163–1184. https://doi:10.1037/a0015738

Roberts, R., Golding, J., Towell, T., and Weinreb, I. (1999). The effects of economic circumstances on British students' mental health. *American College of Health*, 48, 3, 103–109. http://www.ncbi.nlm.nih.gov/pubmed/10584444

Röhricht, F., Sattel, H., Kuhn, C., and Lahmann, C. (2019). Group body psychotherapy for the treatment of somatoform disorder: A partly randomised controlled feasibility pilot study. *BMC Psychiatry*, 19, 120. https://doi.org/10.1186/s12888-019-2095-6

Rosendal, M., Carlsen, A. H., Rask, M. T., and Moth, G. (2015). Symptoms as the main problem in primary care: A cross-sectional study of frequency and characteristics. *Scandinavian Primary Health Care*, 33(2), 91–99. https://doi: 10.3109/02813432.2015.1030166

Sanders, M. (2023). Student Mental Health in 2023 (pp. 24–26). Transforming Access and Student Outcomes in Higher Education. https://www.kcl.ac.uk/policy-institute/assets/student-mental-health-in-2023.pdf

Schneiderman, N., Ironson, G., and Siegel, S. D. (2005). Stress and health: Psychological, behavioural, and biological determinants. *Annual Review of Clinical Psychology*, 1, 607–628. doi:10.1146/annurev.clinpsy.1.102803.144141

Seth, A. K. and Friston, K. J. (2016). Active interoceptive inference and the emotional brain. *Philos. Trans. R. Soc. B Biol. Sci.*, 371:20160007.

Shafir, T. (2015). Movement based strategies for emotion regulation. In M. L. Bryant (Ed.), *Handbook on Emotion Regulation: Processes, Cognitive Effects and Social Consequences* (pp. 231–249). Nova Science Publishers.

Soet, J., and Sevig, T. (2006). Mental health issues facing a diverse sample of college students: results from the college student mental health survey. *NASPA*, 43(3), 410–431, https://doi:10.2202/1949-6605.1676

Stallman, H. M. (2010). Psychological distress in university students: A comparison with general population data. *Australian Psychologist*, 45, 4, 249–257. https://doi.org/10.1080/00050067.2010.482109

Steinbrecher, N., Koerber, S., Frieser, D., and Hiller, W. (2011). The prevalence of medicallyunexplained symptoms in primary care. *Psychosomatics*, 52(3), 263–271. https://doi:10.1016/j.psym.2011.01.007

Stephan, K. E. … and Petzschner, F. H. (2016). Allostatic self-efficacy: A metacognitive theory of dyshomeostasis-induced fatigue and depression. *Front. Hum. Neurosci.*, 15(10), 550.

Stones, S., and Glazzard, J. (2019). *Supporting Student Mental Health in Higher Education.*Critical Publishing.

Student Minds. (2023, February). Student Minds Research Briefing – February 2023.

Student Minds. (2024). The Student Mental Health Manifesto. https://www.studentminds.org.uk/uploads/3/7/8/4/3784584/2024_manifesto_digital_final_high_res.pdf

Sugawara, A. … and Sekiguchi A. (2020). Effects of interoceptive training on decision making, anxiety and somatic symptoms. *Biopsychosoc. Med.*, 17(14), 7.

Thorley, C. (2017). *Not by Degrees: Improving Student Health in the UK's Universities*. Institute for Public Policy Research. www.ippr.org/publications/not-by-degrees

Unite. (2016). *Student resilience: Unite students insight report*. Bristol: Unite Students. Retrieved 14/1/21 from: https://www.unite-group.co.uk/sites/default/files/2017-03/student-insight-report-2016.pdf

Universities UK. (2019). *Step Change.* https://universitiesuk.ac.uk/policy-and-analysis/stepchange/Pages/framework.aspx

University and College Admission Service (UCAS). (2021). *Starting the Conversation: UCAS Report on Student Mental Health*. UCAS.

University College London Union (UCL). (2019). *Heads Up: Reporting on Mental Health*. https://studentsunionucl.org/sites/uclu.org/files/u198046/documents/heads_up_-_reporting_on_mental_health_online_final.pdf

Verger, P., Combes, J., B., … and Perettti-Wattel, P. (2009). Psychological distress in first year university students: socioeconomic, academic stressors, mastery and social support in young men and women. *Social Psychiatry and Psychiatric Epidemiology*, 44(8), 643–650.

Verhaak, P. F., Meijer, S. A., Visser, A. P., Wolters, G. (2006). Persistent presentation of medically unexplained symptoms in general practice. *Family Practice*, 23(4), 414–420. doi: 10.1093/fampra/cml016. Epub 2006 Apr 21. PMID: 16632487

Walsemann, K. M., Gee, G. C., and Gentile, D. (2015). Sick of our loans: student borrowing and the mental health of young adults in the United States. *Social Science and Medicine*, 124, 85–93. doi: 10.1016/j.socscimed.2014.11.027

Weale, S. (2023). High court to consider whether universities owe students legal duty of care. *The Guardian*, November 20. https://shorturl.at/dDhij

Webb, E., Ashton, C. H., Kelly, P. and Kamali, F. (1996). Alcohol and drug use in UK university students. *Lancet*, 348(9032), 922–925. http://www.ncbi.nlm.nih.gov/pubmed/8843811

Williams, M., Coare, P., and Anderson, J. (2015). *Higher Education Funding Council for England* (HEFCE). https://www.employment-studies.co.uk/resource/understanding-provision-students- mental-health-problems-and-intensive-support-needs

YouGov. (2016). One in four students suffer from mental health problems. *YouGov*, August 9. https://yougov.co.uk/society/articles/16156-quarter-britains-students-are-afflicted-mental-hea

Chapter 9

Somatisation, Chronic Stress and The BodyMind Approach

Introduction

People with MUS are difficult to engage with psychological interventions and can feel misunderstood and stigmatised (Blom et al., 2012). The diagnosis as "unexplained" is unhelpful and can lead to further distress and a belief the symptoms are "imagined, feigned or 'all in the mind'" (Brown, 2007, p. 778). Approaches to treatment are generally limited to primary care management and/or psychological methods such as cognitive behaviour therapy (CBT) for some conditions (Kroenke, 2007), which are usually rejected as unacceptable by this population (De Lusignan et al., 2013) possibly due to stigma.

It is acknowledged that MUS is not simply a psychological condition, however the prevalence of treatment with CBT in the National Health Service (NHS) appears to regard it as such. In a study by Andrews et al. (2018) perceiving a psychological cause for MUS was related to more negative health outcomes (moderate to large effect) and more negative emotional coping (small effect). If this is so, then one-to-one psychological therapies such as CBT are less likely to be successful than The BodyMind Approach (TBMA) proposed here, which does not require a psychological explanatory model.

Rubin and Wessely (2006) linked chronic stress to MUS, and MUS is also linked to stress system dysfunction (Luyten et al., 2012). This chapter aims to introduce the reader to an explanation of the physiological mechanisms underlying chronic stress experienced in MUS and which we could also extend to BDD. Furthermore, an approach is explored which enables people with MUS/BDD to learn to self-manage their condition through emotional self-regulation, working through the body. Examples of aspects we believe are responsible for this learning are highlighted.

The BodyMind Approach

The BodyMind Approach is a course of 12 facilitated, experiential, group-work sessions leading to a tailor-made action plan, designed and owned by

DOI: 10.4324/9781003460749-10

the person, with the intention of embedding new self- management learning habits. Learning takes place through interaction with the facilitator trained in TBMA and the group.

For the 2004–08 TBMA study (Payne, 2009a, b; Payne & Stott, 2010) to give the message that the sessions were concerned with personal learning through, and of symptoms, the groups were termed "Learning Groups" to remove the stigma of mental health (the label often given for MUS). Furthermore, this shows a valuing of the body symptoms rather than dismissing them as "all in the mind". This, and the venue being in a community centre, help participants to access the intervention through self-referral (as well as general practitioners [GPs]), especially for those resistant to mental health explanations, psychological therapies and/or the associated stigma.

In TBMA people learn by engaging the body through non-verbal processes and subsequently encompassing the mind (called embodied learning) which, in this case, draws on the body's responses to stress (McCloud, 2010). This learning becomes an iterative process, from body to mind and then mind to body leading to self-management.

For a description of TBMA; its theory, philosophy and content; and the structure of the programme, see Payne and Brooks (2018). (For a review of the literature on the treatment of MUS and how TBMA as discussed below builds on this, see Payne and Brooks, 2016.) Outcomes from data for the effectiveness of TBMA from research and evidence-based practice are detailed in Payne and Stott (2010) and Payne and Brooks (2017). This chapter does not attempt to give a step-by-step account of TBMA, rather it elucidates the mechanisms it is believed are involved in the embodied learning for self-management.

People suffering from MUS/BDD may experience their body as an enemy because of the unpleasant physical sensations of symptoms. Transforming this into seeing the body as something trustworthy is one of the outcomes from TBMA. By listening to their body people learn they can trust their bodies. The BodyMind Approach supports people to learn the connection between physical sensations and emotions (Critchley & Garfinkel, 2017). The development of a benign relationship with the body allows people to take care of themselves by giving it kind attention through the practice of mindfulness through the body (somatic mindfulness), where the focus is on the body rather than the mind. Somatic mindfulness is an alternative to an earlier term "bodymindfulness" (Payne & Brooks, 2017: 65). It concerns the focus of attention and is a specific practice, whereas embodied learning is the outcome of the whole process. Somatic mindfulness is one of the main methodologies of TBMA. The facilitator guides people to develop the capacity to attend to their internal awareness of experience, finding ways to engage with what they notice (often during a movement practice with eyes half closed or closed) internally over several minutes. These practices can be undertaken at home as well as in the group setting. Learning how they are feeling somatically and how to interpret information about sensations promotes self-care. This may also reduce any tendency to catastrophise symptoms. It is a perceptual learning and creative process. Supporting people to connect deeply with their bodies is fundamentally helping them to become aware of bodily sensations through self-massage/touch and mindful attention to interoceptive experience (Craig, 2002).

To experience this sensation as a reader, move and pause and ask yourself of what you are aware? Massage your hand for a few seconds with the other hand and pause, become aware of the sensation. Breathe through the nose and bring kind mindful attention to the breathing, thus engaging with it in a somatic way, noticing the sensations in the body as you breath in and out through the nose.

In TBMA expressive movement is introduced with an internal focus of attention (eyes gazing down or closed – they can be opened at any time), i.e. listening to the bodily sensations as messages to be expressed. This invites consideration of what people might be aware of in their body. Thereafter, expressing the internal experience takes place through, for example, hand gestures. Then participants are invited make marks on paper or write in their journal what they recall of their body speaking, through movement, about their internal subjective experience of the symptoms. Later they may be offered a witness which may support and validate their recall of the gestures, feelings, inner imaginative and bodily felt experience. The witness speaks after the mover and uses self-referential language, owning their own point of view on the impact of the gestures on their being which may or may not validate the mover (if not, it is something they can consider anyway). This is an adapted form of Authentic Movement (Adler, 2002; Payne, 2025). In this way, TBMA helps people with MUS/BDD to develop a language for identifying and becoming aware of bodily sensations from a new, and different perspective. Exercises such as guided movement practices increase the capacity to attend with kind attention to internal experience in the present moment. Supporting people with MUS/BDD to learn to bring a different sort of attention to their bodies can create resistance and fear. Someone who has lived with unexplained pain (e.g. fibromyalgia) for 20 years will have developed coping mechanisms, including medication, which may be hard to shift. They might need to learn in a slow and stepped way to build trust; learning they can connect with their body and be present to it may, at first, be a scary experience.

Self-management is normally regarded as a top-down cognitive approach for people with medical conditions (see Payne & Brooks, 2018, for a rationale for self-management in health education for this population). The authors view TBMA as a bottom-up approach in that it works from the body to the mind, privileging sensory experience, rather than the conventional top-down solely cognitive orientation which privileges will, language and reason for a set of beliefs and emotions. Shapiro (2011) shows us that cognitions start in part as a subjective emotional experience based in the body. This view of TBMA as a bottom-up approach is consistent with notions of self-management, promoting self-care.

TBMA is a bodily re-learning programme, which aims to change responses to symptoms. There are specific aspects of TBMA which facilitate learning which are described below:

a) increasing the capacity to be present in the "here and now" (i.e., maintaining awareness of inner experience without dissociating) during the practices
b) developing body literacy (the ability to identify and articulate bodily experience), learning inner body awareness approaches to facilitate access to somatic and emotional awareness
c) exploring the symptom through the imagination, sensation and its characteristics can bring meaning to the symptom, which may help toward an understanding of its function in day-to-day life
d) verbal processing of the practice experiences facilitates further cognitive understanding and promotes social interaction
e) journaling facilitates learning as participants reflect on their journey, noting insights, strategies for self-management, goals etc.
f) an action plan helps consolidate the learning from these reflections. It is designed, together with the facilitator, during the last individual consultation. The action plan gives a map for self-management acting as a maintenance tool post-group
g) learning is maintained by reminders/nudges sent every six weeks during the six-month post-group phase, nudging people to adhere to the plan, embedding a new habit.

Outcomes from TBMA include the capacity for self-compassion and acceptance as well as insight (Payne & Brooks, 2018). Thus, these practices are thought to facilitate increased body awareness as a primary strategy for dissociation reduction, involving the connection between sensory, emotional and cognitive awareness (Levine, 1997; Ogden & Minton, 2000).

Learning and The BodyMind Approach

Learning for adults with MUS/BDD is essential for new habits to be formed, interrupting the spiralling of old habits leading to anxiety, depression and more severe symptom distress. The BodyMind Approach is research-informed; it is based on embodied social cognition theory (Lindblom, 2015), acknowledged by neuroscience research as the new wave, and enactivism, defined as dynamic interaction between an acting organism and its environment. Davis and Markman (2012) allude to the future of embodied cognition. It appears aspects of cognition are based on sensorimotor circuitry and physical experience to develop and rely on physical involvement for performance.

Enactivism has an antecedent in the work of Bruner (1964), who invented the term. One of the central claims of the "enactive perspective" (Varela, Thompson & Rosch, 1991) concerns the deep continuity between mind and life, where cognition is understood to originate in the self-organising activity of living biological systems (Maturana & Varela, 1980, 1984; Varela, Thompson & Rosch, 1991; Thompson, 2007; Di Paolo, Buhrmann & Barandiaran, 2017). This view of cognition is not wholly driven by the environment, nor by internal representations, but rather by the embodied activity of living agents (brain, body and the environment). Embodied cognition is about acknowledging the roles which perception, action, and the environment play in learning. Consequently, it can be said "embodiment is the surprisingly radical hypothesis the brain is not the sole cognitive resource we have available to us to solve problems" (Wilson & Golonka, 2013, p. 2).

In cognitive science the content of internal cognitive representations is seen as the most important determinant of the structure of our behaviour. Cognitive science identifies this content and how it is accessed and used. However, what has not been accounted for is that we have extremely high-quality access to the environment through perception, which can be an additional resource. Hence, the new wave in cognitive science is the notion that cognition is embodied (Shapiro, 2011; Wilson & Golonka, 2013). From this point of view, if cognition spans brain, body, and the environment (i.e. the mind, Siegal, 2017), then states of mind of a disembodied nature do not exist to be modified. On this view cognition is a comprehensive system pulled together from an extensive range of resources.

Embodied social cognition means "engaging with another as a person involving adopting a personal stance, comprised of affective and bodily relatedness" claims Ratcliffe (2007, p. 23). This author continues to say interpersonal engagement ordinarily is fully embodied, in that communication relies heavily on individuals' postures, gestures and facial expressions. In face-to-face interaction we can perceive another's intention, desires and feelings through participatory sense-making.

TBMA is based on this functional unity of body and mind which have an inter-connected, reciprocal relationship. It recognises that our learning experiences are formed, expressed and reshaped through the body. It is through the body and movement that we experience the world. It is our first learning environment as an infant. TBMA builds on this as a biopsychosocial approach because it is holistic and integrates body (bio) and mind (psyche) in a group (social) setting. In TBMA it is by learning through the body experience that chronic stress is alleviated. Furthermore, it encompasses the participant's personal social situation when they are exploring and learning about their symptoms and how to self-manage them in TBMA.

At the forefront of this learning approach is a pre-occupation with the body often experienced by people with MUS. This focus is harnessed to foster curiosity about symptoms and their possible management through TBMA. Experimentation through sensory perception and physical impulses expressed as movement in whole or parts of the body becomes possible.

This can help access the roots of previous experience in the lived body, as well as access to autonomic impulses and pre-lingual processes. Thus, it can become a platform for the formation of meaning-making in relation to symptoms which, to date, have eluded an explanation by both the medical profession and the person concerned.

The Importance of the Chronic Stress Response in Medically Unexplained Symptoms/Body Distress Disorder and Its Interruption by The BodyMind Approach

Emotions being stuck in a previously formed habit as a response to chronic stress does not comprise a psychological condition in the authors' view. MUS/BDD can both be seen as an emotional condition rather than simply a psychological one. However, the stress response can be a useful explanation for, and a way of working with, symptoms.

We propose a theory of how TBMA works below. A theory is a "… statement of concepts and their interrelationships that shows how and/or why a phenomenon occurs" (Corley & Gioia, 2011, p. 12). Connections may be made between the stress responses in the body (the symptom) and co-occurring emotional distress conditions such as depression, anxiety etc., in MUS/BDD. The importance of thoughts and emotions as fleeting, changing in dynamic ways, is that they are only a reality in the moment, whereas the sensory experience of MUS/BDD is in the body and experienced over time.

Thoughts and feelings are interpretations in response to the body-felt experience in the environment. Since emotions are embodied, they can get stuck as sensory experiences and thus be held onto rather than experienced as passing through. Additionally, every time a similar emotion is stimulated it travels the same pathway routinely and the sensation persists. These sensations can therefore become physically maintained over time (chronic). However, it is possible to interrupt the cycle by re-interpreting and re-framing the sensory experience to enhance a more positive experience. The BodyMind Approach offers experiential "practices" which enable the participant to, for example, concentrate on "well" areas of the body, learn the signals in the body for chronic stress and wellbeing and use their imagination to tap into the unconscious aspects of the symptom. These help them to gain an understanding of the gains and losses involved in the persistence of the symptom, and an opportunity to re-frame the symptom and its function. The knowledge of self which is gained from these experiences culminates in what appears to be an increased capacity to self-manage (Payne & Brooks, 2017).

For people with MUS/BDD, in addition to symptoms being a possible response to excessive pressure, there is distress from the anticipation and experience of the symptoms themselves. There is a greater focus on the body, hypervigilant monitoring of bodily signals, and self-focusing (as in hypochondriasis). The body becomes viewed by the patient as alarmingly problematic rather than being the subject of perception in a non-judgmental, accepting way. This hypervigilance exacerbates the symptom distress leading to a distancing from the body (dissociation), whereby the body becomes the enemy. There is then a need to protect themselves rather than sensations being part of the background of the embodied experience of the world, "leaving the individual without bodily based emotional tools for self-regulation processes" (Damasio, 2005, cited in Valenzuela-Moguillansky, Reyes-Reyes& Gaete, 2018, p. 115). The BodyMind Approach reverses this situation whereby the person becomes friendly towards their symptom and begins to see it as an ally (Ataria, 2016) in highlighting the need for self-regulation. This achieves a re-connection with the body and sensations rather than a distancing, resulting in body compassion. Learning from the symptom can inform the person when they are out of balance, thus helping them to take steps to re-balance (valuing the body and its signals). People learn there is no need to attempt to banish the symptom but to reframe perception. The symptom can even be welcomed as an early warning signal for self-care action, i.e. to be able to cope – an empowering experience enabling the person to take back control. The focus is on living well by regulating symptoms rather than a cure or treatment.

Homeostatic Regulation

Figure 9.1 shows how the stress response resolves under normal circumstances. A stimulus can create a somatic experience which is then interpreted, depending on its threat level, to which a reaction then occurs. Under normal circumstances noradrenalin, adrenalin and cortisol (see Figure 9.1) are produced, leading to a mobility or immobility stress response. Their production and effects are normally fleeting, being used to resolve the threat situation.

Figure 9.2 below provides an overview of the mechanism at work in the body when the threat is internal, persistent and unresolved. This results in a positive feedback loop maintaining the symptom distress which gets increasingly out of control. In MUS/BDD, adrenaline and cortisol are produced (see Figure 9.2) constantly due to the nature of the threat to wellbeing in the body itself which is unresolvable.

Consequently, the unexplained symptoms originating from external environmental stressors (such as workplace stress) which are also unresolvable, become chronic. The symptom is experienced as an internal threat to wellbeing provoking and/or constantly maintaining the stress response, leading to

corrective mechanism resolves threat (flight-fight-freeze-faint-fold)

Anxiety/fear

Anxiety/fear

Threat

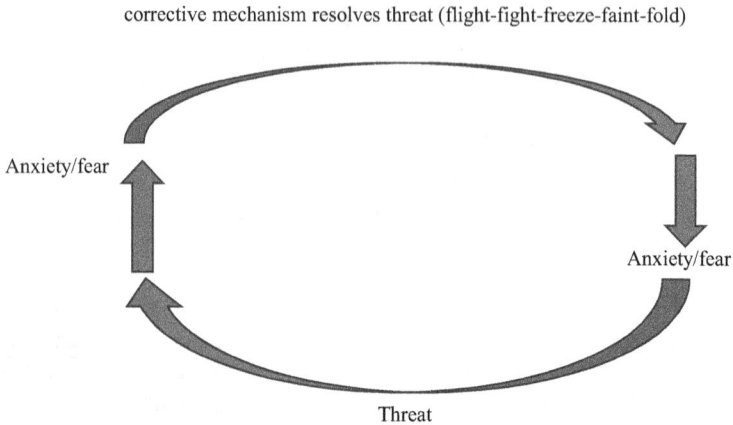

Figure 9.1   A negative feedback (corrective) loop: homeostasis working correctly

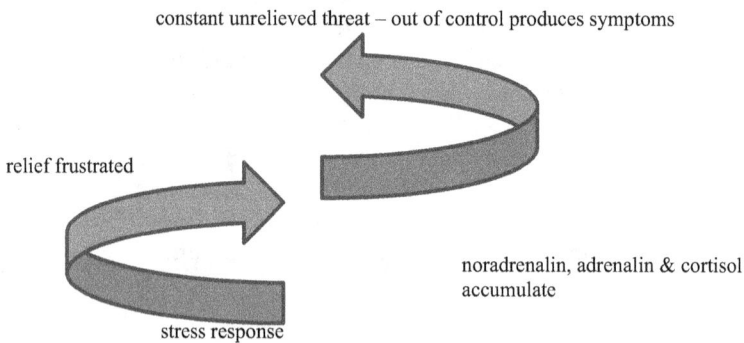

constant unrelieved threat – out of control produces symptoms

relief frustrated

noradrenalin, adrenalin & cortisol accumulate

stress response

Figure 9.2   A positive feedback loop – a spiral

either mobility or immobility. In the case of the stress response of immobility (faint, fold) due to the excessive cortisol, the musculature collapses leading to flaccidity can be interpreted as, or exacerbate, depression. Alternatively, the threat response of immobility may lead to tetany leading to rigidity. This can be viewed as the freeze or fold stress response manifested as total shut down emotionally, another form of depression, or possibly disconnecting from the body, feelings, thoughts etc. in a form of dissociation and/or alexithymia.

Anxiety may be linked to the threat response of mobility (fight, flight) which cannot be resolved. When anxious, our bodies secrete adrenalin and cortisol, which prepare the body for flight or fight by increasing heart rate and blood pressure and diverting blood away from the gut (slowing down digestion) to the muscles. In some stressful situations it is often impossible (when an infant, for example) or inappropriate (for example, at work) to fight or run away, so the situation remains unresolved and therefore the body responses are perpetuated. The experience is of chronic anxiety at various levels, which never gets turned off. The physiological happenings in the body, for example, a constant tetanic muscle response to anxiety, can lead to pain and inflammation such as found in fibromyalgia.

Paradoxically, tests and scans come back negative in MUS, and in theory should be reassuring, but actually lead to hyper-arousal and catastrophising because of the body-felt experience convincing the sufferer there is some-thing wrong. Anxiety is increased, contributing to a chronic condition. The fact that it cannot be found is therefore no comfort but leads to requests for further investigation. Because the stress response cannot be acted on (by, for example, running away, or standing to fight), the response becomes stuck or chronic. A positive feedback loop is created which increases distress even further. As other stressful, threatening situations occur, which they do in life, such as complex bereavement, trauma, domestic violence or substance abuse, the pattern of response to stress is repeated forming habitual behaviour.

TBMA is a supportive, facilitated, interactive groupwork programme employing experimental play with the symptom through movement and the body. Porges' Polyvagal Theory concludes that human social interaction combined with taking the psychological mind-set into account in interven-tions turns off the sympathetic fight/flight response. The calming of the sym-pathetic system, together with feeling listened to in the group, enables people to feel safe enough to engage in self-reflection with the group to achieve self-regulation and self-management (Porges, 2003)

In Figure 9.3 the negative feedback loop is restored as people learn how to self-manage. Initially symptoms may be a result of a culmination of

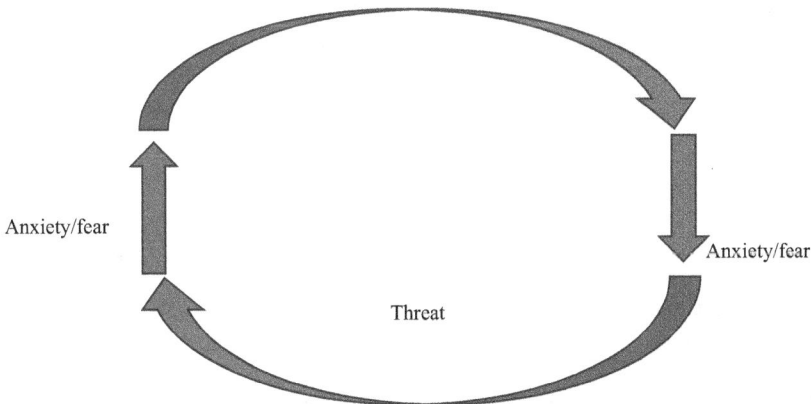

Figure 9.3   TBMA substituting for the natural resolution

unresolved stress responses leading to a breakdown of homeostasis (a lack of self-regulation, as in Figure 9.2). TBMA helps to restore a homeostatic feedback loop for correction using tools (i.e. skills, strategies, processes) learned to enable the tactics required for self-regulation. These tactics can be employed at any time in a self-management strategy which interrupts the unresolved stress response positive feedback loop. Hence, the importance of TBMA introducing tools which facilitate learning self-management is clear.

Summary

Using research from embodied social cognition, TBMA appears to offer an avenue for learning to self-manage. The interruption of the chronic stress response afforded by the learning in TBMA may provide an explanatory model for MUS helping sufferers and health professionals understand this, as yet unexplained, condition. It gives a start to making sense of the connections between body and mind as manifested in an organically unexplained symptom. Furthermore, our experience of delivering TBMA suggests that people with MUS find this explanation acceptable. They report they learned about more links between body and mind and have greater awareness of these connections (Payne & Brooks, 2018).

References

Adler, J. (2002). *Offering from the Conscious Body: The Discipline of Authentic Movement*. Inner Traditions.

Ataria, Y. (2016). When the body becomes the enemy: Disownership toward the body. *Philosophy, Psychiatry, and Psychology*, 23(1), 1–15. https://doi.org/10.1353/ppp.2016.0002

Blom, D., Thomaes, S., ... and Geenen, R. (2012). A combination of illness invalidation from the work environment and helplessness is associated with embitterment in patients with FM. *Rheumatology*, 51, 347–353. https://doi.org/10.1093/rheumatology/ker342

Brown, R. J. (2007). Introduction to the special issue on medically unexplained symptoms: background and future directions. *Clinical Psychology Review*, 27, 769–780. https://doi.org/10.1016/j.cpr.2007.07.003

Bruner, J. S. (1964). The course of cognitive growth. *American Psychologist*, 19, 1–15. doi: 10.1037/h0044160

Corley, K. G., and Gioia, D. A. (2011). Building theory about theory building: what constitutes a theoretical contribution? *Academy of Management Review*, 36(1), 12–32.

Craig, A. D. (2002). How do you feel? Interoception: the sense of the physiological condition of the body. *Nature Reviews Neuroscience*, 3 (8): 655–666. doi:10.1038/nrn894.

Critchley, H. D., and Garfinkel, S. N. (2017). Interoception and emotion. *Current Opinion in Psychology*, 17, 7–14.

Davis, J. I., and Markman, A. B. (2012). Embodied cognition as a practical paradigm: introduction to the topic, the future of embodied cognition. *Topics in Cognitive Science*, 4(4), 685–691.

Damasio, A. (2005). *Descartes' Error: Emotion, Reason, and the Human Brain* (Reprint edition). Penguin Books.

De Lusignan, S., Jones, S., ... and Chan, T. (Eds.) (2013). IAPT LTC/MUS Pathfinder evaluation project phase 1 Final Report, November 2013 (Revised April 2014). University of Surrey Evaluation Team, University of Surrey.

Di Paolo, E. A., Buhrmann, T., and Barandiaran, X. E. (2017). *Sensorimotor Life: An Enactive Proposal*. Oxford University Press.

Kroenke, K. (2007). Efficacy of treatment for somatoform disorders: A review of randomized controlled trials. *Psychosomatic Medicine*, 69, 881–888. https://doi.org/10.1097/PSY.0b013e 31815b00c4

Levine, P. (1997). *Waking the Tiger: Healing Trauma*. North Atlantic Books.

Lindblom, J. (2015). *Embodied Social Cognition*. Springer. eBook. Doi:10.1007/978-3-319-20315-7

Luyten, P., van Houdenhove, B., ... and Fonagy, P. (2012). A mentalization based approach to the understanding and treatment of functional somatic disorders. *Psychoanalytic Psychotherapy*, 26(2), 121–140. https://doi.org/10.1080/02668 734.2012.678061

Maturana, H. (1991). Science and daily life: the ontology of scientific explanations, In F. Steier (Ed.), *Research and Reflexivity* (pp. 30–52). Sage.

Maturana, H., and Varela, F. (1980). *Autopoiesis and Cognition: The Realization of the Living*. Reidel.

Maturana, H., and Varela, F. (1984). *The Tree of Knowledge: The Biological Roots of Human Understanding*. New Science Library.

McAndrew L. M., Crede, M., ... Phillips, L. A. (2018). Using the common-sense model to understand health outcomes for medically unexplained symptoms: a meta-analysis. *Health Psychology Review*, 9, 1–20. doi: 10.1080/17437199.2018.1521730.

McLeod, S. A. (2010). What is the stress response. Retrieved from https://www.simpl ypsychology.org/stress-biology.html

Ogden, P., and Minton, K. (2000). Sensorimotor psychotherapy: one method for processing traumatic memory. *Traumatology*, 6(3), 149–173.

Payne, H. (2009a). The BodyMind Approach to psychotherapeutic groupwork with patients with medically unexplained symptoms: a review of the literature, description of approach and methodology selected for a pilot study. *European Journal for Counselling and Psychotherapy*, 11, 3, 287–310.

Payne, H. (2009b). Pilot study to evaluate Dance Movement Psychotherapy (the BodyMind Approach) with patients with medically unexplained symptoms: participant and facilitator perceptions and a summary discussion. *Int. Journal for Body, Movement and Dance in Psychotherapy*, 5, 2, 95–106.

Payne, H. (2025). *Authentic Movement: A Culmination of Theory, Research and Practice*. Routledge.

Payne, H., and Brooks, S. (2016). Clinical outcomes and cost benefits from The BodyMind Approach™ for Patients with Medically Unexplained Symptoms in Primary Health Care in England: Practice-Based Evidence. *Arts in Psychotherapy*, 47, 55–65.

Payne, H., and Brooks, S. (2017). Moving on: The BodyMind Approach™ for medically unexplained symptoms. *Public Mental Health Journal*, 10, 2.

Payne, H., and Brooks, S (2018). Different Strokes for Different Folks: The BodyMind Approach as a Learning Tool for Patients With Medically Unexplained Symptoms to Self-Manage. Front. Psychol. 9:2222. doi: 10.3389/fpsyg.2018.02222

Payne, H., and Brooks, S. (2020). A theory of learning for self-management: A qualitative analysis of patient perceptions of The BodyMind Approach™ for people with medically unexplained symptoms. *Front. Psychol.*, 07 December 2020, Sec. *Health Psychology*, 11 – 2020 | https://doi.org/10.3389/fpsyg.2020.554566

Payne, H. and Stott, D. (2010). Change in the moving bodymind: Quantitative results from a pilot study on the BodyMind Approach (BMA) as groupwork for patients with medically unexplained symptoms (MUS). *Counselling and Psychotherapy Research*, 10,4, 295–307.

Porges, S. (2003). Social engagement and attachment: A phylogenetic perspective. *Annals of New York Academy of Sciences*, 1008, 31–47.

Ratcliffe, M. (2007). *Rethinking Commonsense Psychology*. Palgrave Macmillan.

Rubin, J., and Wessely, S. (2006). The role of stress in the etiology of medically unexplained syndromes. In B. B. Arnetz and R. Ekman (Eds.), *Stress in Health and Disease* (pp. 292–306). Wiley-VCH Verlag GmbH and Co KGaA. https://doi.org/10.1002/3527609156

Shapiro, L. (2011) *Embodied Cognition*. Routledge Press.

Thompson, E. (2007). *Mind in Life: Biology, Phenomenology, and the Sciences of Mind*. Harvard University Press.

Valenzuela-Moguillansky, C., Reyes-Reyes, A., and Gaete, M. I. (2018). Exteroceptive and interoceptive body-self-awareness in fibromyalgia patients. In: M. Sestito., A. Raballo., G. Stanghellini and V. Gallese. (Eds), Editorial: Embodying the Self: Neurophysiological Perspectives on the Psychopathology of Anomalous Bodily Experiences. *Frontiers in Human Neuroscience* (pp. 114–28). doi: 10.3389/978-2-88945-456-3

Varela, F., Thompson, E., and Rosch, E. (1991). *The Embodied Mind: Cognitive Science and Human Experience*. MIT Press.

Wilson, A. D., and Golonka, S. (2013). Embodied cognition is not what you think it is. *Frontiers in Psychology*, 4:58. doi: 10.3389/fpsyg.2013.00058

Chapter 10

Epilogue

Introduction

This chapter provides an overview of all the chapters in the book. It draws out some key underpinnings and provides commentary on the content of these. Furthermore, it offers some thoughts on the future of TBMA, the research and suggestions for practitioners to take TBMA forward in their respective health systems or privately. For patients experiencing MUS the intervention may offer hope for the future as it would for practitioners.

Overview of Chapters

The book begins by introducing the reader to TBMA, how it developed, has been designed and discusses its relevance to BDD including specifically MUS. There is a brief definition of TBMA, MUS and BDD and an outline of the book's content, its audience and how to use it. The chapter also contains previously published material on the learning model for TBMA, comprising adult learning theory (and the Johari Window), transformational and experiential learning.

Chapter 2 provides brief historical synthesis of the terms employed for bodily symptoms for which tests and scans all come back negative. Following this, the research into MUS – before the term BDD became current – is presented. In Chapter 3 there is additional information with reference to the background and the development of TBMA. The chapter provides a section on self-management, and a discussion of TBMA's theoretical formulation, principles, aims and underlying philosophy. The notion of self-management for the MUS population is explored and the biopsychosocial model highlighted. The importance of bridging the dualistic approach to health is discussed, as is tracking the principles for effective practice with this population. Finally, there is a comparative economic analysis between CBT and TBMA. In Chapter 4 a discussion on TBMA as a group intervention is presented. The programme administration is described, including an overview for delivery. Examples of self- and health professional referral forms are given

DOI: 10.4324/9781003460749-11

for reference, together with the inclusion and exclusion criteria for the selection of participants derived from previous research. Both the intake and exit individual meetings are explained. There is an example of programme content for each of the 12 sessions, a session example and an overview of the five phases of a session.

Chapter 5 covers the training of TBMA group facilitators. The prerequisites for candidates training in TBMA, the content of training modules and the assessments are provided. Information distributed during the training, the attitude of mind expected of facilitators and guidance on the facilitation of the groups are included. The attributes, skills, knowledge and understanding of facilitators are itemised. The need for boundaries and the role of the facilitator are identified and explanatory points to give to health professionals and group participants supplied. A suggested disclaimer statement of understanding for participants is also given. Both GP/commissioners and participant/patient exemplar brochures which explain the groups are included. Additionally, suggested examples of forms for use by the facilitator include a patient self-referral form, an accident and incident form and an attendance recording form. Finally, an example of the local and national resources list which facilitators could give to group participants at the end of their TBMA course is proposed.

Chapter 6 is an updated version of a previously published report of a qualitative study to discover participants' perceptions of the experience of TBMA. The thematic analysis of the data notes five consistent key principles: a) body with mind connections; b) the importance of the facilitator; c) positive benefits; d) preparedness change; and e) acceptance/compassion. These all appear to have kickstarted the self-management process for participants. The perceptions arose from open-ended questions about the programme which did not spotlight the arts/expressive movement practices per se, collected independently from the group and researchers or facilitators, and focused on the group experience. However, because the practices were integral to the group process it is reasonable to infer the perceptions reported connected to these practices. It seems likely, therefore, due to the holistic, integrative nature of TBMA, that all these elements may be involved. Chapter 7 is an amended and updated version of a previously published article in which it is hypothesised that TBMA can support people with insecure attachment styles and MUS to self-manage. This article has illustrated how the design of TBMA is built on the three insecure adult attachment styles associated with MUS. It goes on to explain how TBMA helps people with MUS and insecure attachment styles to learn to self-manage.

In Chapter 8 an argument is made for incorporating workshops in TBMA for students in higher education providers (HEPs). Stones and Glazzard (2019) recommend an institution-wide approach to eradicate stigma toward mental health, one that enables students to be mentally healthy and extends beyond provisions targeting solely mental ill-health. TBMA fits into this extended provision. There are overlaps between the body, mind and aspects of wellbeing (Checkoway, 2011). These overlaps could be captured by TBMA at times of increased stress such as at induction, before/after transitions, placements, examinations and assignment deadlines. TBMA may reduce stigma and attend to students' physical (i.e. bodily symptoms) and emotional distress as part of an overall mental health and wellbeing strategy based in student services/faculties/schools. There are unique opportunities now with the UK University Mental Health Charter (Hughes & Spanner, 2019) to review the way student mental health is regarded, and which evidence-based interventions are accessible and acceptable to all students, not only the minority who are able to engage with student wellbeing services.

Chapter 9 explores the relationship between TBMA, MUS/BDD and the stress-response. Research from embodied social cognition appears to offer an avenue for learning to self-manage. The interruption of the chronic stress response afforded by the learning in TBMA may provide an explanatory model for MUS (and, in certain circumstances, depending on the physical diagnosis, BDD), helping sufferers and health professionals understand this unexplained medical condition. It gives a start to making sense of the connections between body and mind as manifested in an organically unexplained symptom. Furthermore, our experience of delivering TBMA suggests that people with MUS find this explanation acceptable. They report they learned about more links between body and mind and have greater awareness of these connections (Payne & Brooks, 2020).

Some Key Underpinnings

Reflecting on these chapters we notice some key underpinnings which contribute to the effectiveness of TBMA. These are not shared in the totality with other interventions for MUS, indeed some may not appear in any such interventions. As such, TBMA forms a unique approach to supporting people experiencing MUS.

Firstly, TBMA is more widely accepted due to it being promoted as a class/workshop called, for example, "Learning About Your Symptoms Group" when people, including students, are resistant to the offer of mental health interventions (such as CBT, counselling/psychotherapy) due to stigma. This is important to ensure people not only start TBMA but maintain their attendance. This is also aided by the friendships that start to form as they share this group activity. Acceptability of the programme by the participant thus reduces attrition which helps the group to feel safe and secure. It also largely enables participants to engage fully in the activities/practices offered. The notion of the programme being a learning process helps with acceptability. This acceptance by participants also decreases the medicalisation of the symptom, normalising it.

There is also the notion of belonging to a group with a common understanding and purpose which reduces the sense of isolation for people with MUS/BDD. They also make friends in the groups. The stigma and shame linked to their symptoms is thus reduced. The feeling of belonging reduces stress and aids wellbeing. Self-confidence, self-esteem and self-respect can be boosted by the feeling of belonging. It also helps safeness and hopefulness for change. This approach has these factors in common with other group approaches such as coercive control and substance abuse groups. This sense of belonging combats their usual feelings of isolation which inhibits the self-confidence and the capacity for change which people with MUS/BDD can experience.

The "biopsychosocial" concept is fully embraced by TBMA, meaning participants in the programme are seen holistically, the intervention fitting the person and group rather than a manualised set of uniform practices in a prescriptive format into which the recipient must fit. Participants do not have to make their symptom known in the group and therefore they are not stigmatised as the problem-symptom or labelled as a particular medical specialism. People are therefore not reduced to their symptom, which is only one part of them, but seen as a whole person with sensory experiences in their whole body. In this way, it obviates the need for the physical problem to be a solely physical problem, allowing it to arise from the complexity of the biopsychosocial environment. Taking the symptom as a gateway to the mind frees the mind to consider other possible causes, and hence opens-up creative options, management, actions etc. The biopsychosocial approach fits synergistically with a group format. It brings about a richness of options from others and the interactive practices.

Another key point might be that TBMA can be made accessible to anyone. This refers to its availability, for example, to welcome self-referrals (with GP agreement of suitability) and to be held in a local community venue. Referral does not have to be via a health professional, nor does it need to be delivered in a health/medical setting. This fits politically with the current governmental changes in the UK, where self-responsibility and prevention in the community is emphasised in healthcare. The programme invites people with a range of symptoms, and more than one. Groups are heterogeneous as opposed to only recruiting participants who have the same symptom. This also allows for richness of experience and changes in behaviour (especially self-management), even though the symptom is not necessarily known to everyone in the group. The venue being based in the community, local to participants also offers accessibility and removes the stigma of attending mental health venues.

The programme is designed with insecure adult attachment styles in mind. We have leaned heavily on Adshead and Guthrie (2015) for the basis of this conceptual framework. Insecure attachment may reduce the motivation for some participants. They may not trust the facilitator and/or others in the group, or they may believe in a magical cure. Others may require constant reassurance from both group and facilitator. Some insecure attachment styles may be unable to sustain any type of intervention. At each stage of the programme insecure attachment styles have been addressed and facilitators are trained to recognise these styles and take account of them in their facilitation. The structure of the programme takes account of these styles – for example, commitment can be for six sessions only at the outset, giving an escape route if needed. In fact, participants, by that stage, do not wish to leave in general. There is also the front loading for the first four sessions (twice a week) to generate group bonding/cohesion and intake meetings with the facilitator to create a relationship of safety.

The fundamental approach in TBMA is based on adult learning theory which supports the accessibility notion of TBMA, as well as its acceptability. The fact that TBMA is promoted as a learning group, employing experiential learning for self-management, invites participants to consider it non-threatening. In CBT there is clearly learning happening, but it is never acknowledged as such and fails to support itself by referring to adult learning theory. However, learning is not solely cognitive, there is also embodied and kinaesthetic learning. Exploring bodily sensations through experiential learning practices can stimulate cognition and self-awareness to result in new understanding and from this, new actions for self-management. There is a difference between knowing something intellectually and applying something learned from experience in the BodyMind. Thus, all resulting action plans for self-management are tailor-made to reflect the insights and experiences learned by each individual participant. Most people experiencing MUS/BDD are under considerable stress which makes cognitive approaches more difficult to access as the frontal lobe for thinking processes is inhibited. Employing creative, movement experiences can elicit a different sort of knowing from the body which is outside of cognition. Additionally, we know movement whether creative or objective, as in exercise, reduces stress and promotes happy hormones/wellbeing.

The importance of self-management in health is increasingly being promoted in the UK health service. This fits with the fact that TBMA supports self-management of symptoms so participants can live well despite them, albeit with reduced distress. This is crucial in the light of the growing self-management strain in the UK National Health Service. Participants are made aware the programme is to enrich self-management and not to expect it as a treatment or cure. Having said that the research showed symptoms did disappear for some people, and for others the distress was reduced significantly. This provides for a sense of hope for the future. The notion of hope for change is promoted throughout the programme, providing the participant engages with the process. There have been examples of participants resisting the approach in the first few sessions but by the end they are convinced of its effectiveness.

Future Research

Researching TBMA in a new context, such as higher education with students, to see if any differences in outcomes occur for MUS/BDD sufferers, and to explore the referral system and the acceptance/accessibility of TBMA for this population to see whether they differ from TBMA delivery in the health service, is important.

There is also a gap in the service for children and adolescents with unexplained symptoms and health anxiety, for example, abdominal paid or headaches. Schools and special education/pupil referral units etc., could be another context for research.

The programme could be researched with adults or children with explained medical conditions and for whom the degree of distress is excessive, as in BDD. We know there is a strong link between chronic stress and physical conditions so TBMA may offer some support to reducing stress and the self-management of it.

The hypothesis that TBMA can address insecure attachment in people with MUS could be tested in the framework of current knowledge by conducting an adult attachment assessment (Bartholomew & Shaver, 1998) pre- and post-intervention with participants suffering MUS undergoing TBMA.

Research into different ethnicities presenting with symptoms is another area which needs exploration as we know ethnic minorities experience more stress and mental health concerns than their white counterparts.

Suggestions for Practitioners

Here are some suggestions for practitioners to take TBMA forward in their respective health systems or privately. For example, collaborating with other practitioners to approach the health service contractor to fund a pilot TBMA group and evaluate the outcomes.

Also, collaborate with alternative/complementary health practitioners to receive referrals for private patients to form a TBMA group. For example, if they have found difficulties in treating MUS/BDD patients, so as not be seen as a competitor.

If employed in higher education wellbeing/counselling services, TBMA can be incorporated as a triage pathway for students experiencing MUS/BDD.

Hope for the Future

It is hoped that this book will encourage suitably qualified practitioners to access the training and thus spread TBMA across cultures and countries. With more TBMA trained facilitators, more people experiencing MUS could benefit from the approach. This could be in a group and/or individually, either privately or as part of the country's health service/insurance etc.

We hope that the UK NHS might adopt TBMA deliveries once again. With the new reform initiative for NHS and the emphasis on prevention, TBMA could be another tool in the box at primary care level. This intervention prevents patients from being caught up multiple times going to various clinics for investigations, and their GP for referrals, even though they have been before, and an organic cause has already been ruled out (for MUS solely).

For suitably qualified practitioners TBMA training offers another tool in their portfolio. The professional associations for dance movement psychotherapy/therapy and/or body psychotherapy could offer TBMA training as CPD for their members, giving them another string to their bow.

We look forward to hearing from you, the reader, as to how this book has impacted you, and/or supported and stimulated your thinking and practice. Please let us know if you have any ideas going forward.

References

Adshead, G. and Guthrie, E. (2015). The role of attachment in medically unexplained symptoms and long-term illness. *British Journal of Psychological Advances*, 21(3), 167–174.

Bartholomew, K., and Shaver, P. R. (1998). Methods of assessing adult attachment: Do they converge? In J. A. Simpson and W. S. Rholes (Eds.), *Attachment Theory and Close Relationships* (pp. 25–45). The Guilford Press.

Checkoway, B. (2011). New perspectives on civic engagement and psychosocial well-being. *Liberal Education*, 97(2), 6–11.

Hughes, G., and Spanner, L. (2019). *The University Mental Health Charter*. Student Minds.

Payne, H., and Brooks, S. D. (2020). A qualitative study of the views of patients with medically unexplained symptoms on The BodyMind Approach: Employing embodied methods and arts practices for self-management. *Frontiers in Psychology*, 11:554566. doi: 10.3389/fpsyg.2020.554566.

Stones, S., and Glazzard, J. (2019). *Supporting Student Mental Health in Higher Education*. Critical Publishing.

Appendix

List of Synonyms for Medically Unexplained Symptoms/Body Distress Disorder

Body Distress Disorder (BDD)
This is a persistent bodily complaint for which adequate examination (including investigations) does not reveal any specified pathology. MUS/BDD are both terms used to address disorders where physical symptoms have no medical explanation. This concept derives from empirical studies and seems to capture most patients with somatoform disorders and functional somatic syndromes (e.g., fibromyalgia, chronic fatigue syndrome and irritable bowel syndrome).

Conversion Disorder (Functional Neurological Symptom Disorder)
A condition where psychological stress or trauma leads to neurological symptoms such as paralysis, blindness or seizures, with no identifiable medical cause. Conversion disorder is one subtype of MUS.

Frequent Fliers
Used by GPs to describe patients who keep returning regularly to the surgery. Super-users or high utilizers are terms used interchangeably for individuals who visit the health services repeatedly, accounting for disproportionate costs.

Functional Disorders
Conditions in which the normal function of a bodily system is disrupted, but without detectable structural or biochemical abnormalities. Common functional disorders include irritable bowel syndrome (IBS) and fibromyalgia.

Functional Somatic Syndromes (FSS)
A term used to describe a group of disorders, including fibromyalgia, chronic fatigue syndrome and irritable bowel syndrome, that share common features of MUS without clear medical pathology.

Health Anxiety
Excessive worry or fear about having a serious medical condition, often despite reassurance from doctors. Individuals with MUS may also have health anxiety, leading to ongoing concerns about their unexplained symptoms.

Hypochondriasis
An outdated term (or hypochondria/hypochondriac), hypochondriasis is a condition in which a person is excessively and unduly worried about having a serious illness. Hypochondria is an old concept whose meaning has repeatedly changed over its lifespan. It has often been used to dismiss women with anxiety about their health.

Malingerer
A person who pretends to be ill to avoid having to work.

Medically Unexplained Symptoms (MUS)
Physical symptoms for which no clear or consistent medical cause can be identified, despite thorough medical investigation. These symptoms often include pain, fatigue or gastrointestinal issues.

Medically Unexplained Physical Symptoms
Physical symptoms which trigger the sufferer to seek health care, but which remain unexplained after appropriate medical assessment. They are very common and cause significant distress and disability.

Psychosomatic
Relating to the interaction between mind and body, where emotional or psychological factors contribute to physical symptoms. MUS are often considered psychosomatic in nature, as emotional distress can manifest physically.

Somatic Symptom Disorder (SSD)
A mental health disorder characterized by excessive focus on physical symptoms, which may or may not have a medical explanation. SSD can overlap with MUS when the patient experiences significant distress about unexplained symptoms.

Somatization
The tendency to experience and communicate psychological distress through physical symptoms. Somatization is a common phenomenon in MUS, where emotional or mental stress leads to unexplained physical discomfort.

Somatoform Disorders
A group of psychiatric disorders in which patients experience physical symptoms that are inconsistent with or cannot be fully explained by medical conditions. MUS is often associated with somatoform disorders.

List of Abbreviations

ACEs	Adverse childhood experiences
AM	Authentic movement
BDD	Body distress disorder
CBT	Cognitive behaviour therapy
GP	General Practitioner
HEI	Higher education institute
HEP	Higher education provider
IBS	Irritable bowel syndrome
MUS	Medically unexplained symptoms
NHS	National Health Service
OfS	Office for students
TBMA	The BodyMind Approach

Glossary of Terms

Here is a glossary of key terms and definitions related to The BodyMind Approach and medically explained and unexplained symptoms and the associated extreme anxiety.

Action Plan The plan made by participants towards the end of the programme identifying what they will do and when to manage their symptoms for the forthcoming six months and beyond. This plan is derived from their learning during the practices.

Adult Learning Adult learning utilises past life experiences and current understanding of a subject as they learn. It needs to be problem-centred, making the impact more focused on current events or real life.

Agency This refers to the sense of control people feel over their life, their capacity to influence thoughts and behaviour, and have faith in their ability to handle a wide range of tasks and situations. Their sense of agency helps them to be psychologically stable, yet flexible in the face of conflict or change.

Alexithymia Difficulty in recognising or expressing emotions, which may lead to physical symptoms as a way of manifesting psychological distress. Individuals with MUS may have higher levels of alexithymia, complicating their ability to link physical symptoms to emotional states.

Anxiety This is a feeling of fear, dread and uneasiness. It might cause perspiration, restlessness and tension, and a rapid heartbeat. It can be a normal reaction to stress. For example, feeling anxious when faced with a difficult problem at work, before taking a test or before making an important decision.

Attachment This refers to the emotional bond an infant and primary caregiver (such as a mother) form together, especially when viewed as a basis for normal emotional and social development.

Attunement The process of becoming sensitively aware and responsive to one's own bodily signals or to the emotional and physical states of others. TBMA emphasises attunement to the body as a way to understand and regulate emotional experiences.

Biopsychosocial Model A holistic approach to understanding illness that considers biological, psychological and social factors. This model is often applied to MUS, recognising that multiple factors contribute to the experience of symptoms.

BodyMind The integrated concept of the body and mind as interconnected entities that influence each other. In TBMA, the body and mind are viewed as a unified system where physical, emotional and mental experiences are linked.

Bodymindfulness This term adopted by the authors to describe the meeting of bodyfulness with mindfulness which TBMA promotes through various practices.

Conversion Disorder (Functional Neurological Symptom Disorder) A condition where psychological stress or trauma leads to neurological symptoms such as paralysis, blindness or seizures, with no identifiable medical cause. Conversion disorder is one subtype of MUS.

Depression A common mental health condition that can happen to anyone. It is characterised by a low mood and/or loss of pleasure or interest in activities for long periods of time. This is different from regular mood changes and feelings about everyday life.

Embodiment The process of fully experiencing and inhabiting the body in the present moment. In TBMA, embodiment refers to becoming more attuned to bodily sensations and using this awareness to process emotions and thoughts.

Emotional Dysregulation Difficulty in managing or responding appropriately to emotional experiences, which can lead to heightened physical symptoms. Emotional dysregulation is often seen in patients with MUS, where unprocessed emotions manifest as physical complaints.

Expressive Movement The use of physical movement as a form of expression, helping to release emotional tension or communicate nonverbally. In TBMA, expressive movement is used as a therapeutic tool to explore and process emotions.

Facilitator This is the name of the professional who leads The BodyMind Approach programme. They will have been trained and assessed prior to becoming a facilitator for TBMA groups.

Functional Disorders Conditions in which the normal function of a bodily system is disrupted, but without detectable structural or biochemical abnormalities. Common functional disorders include irritable bowel syndrome (IBS) and fibromyalgia.

Functional Somatic Syndromes (FSS) A term used to describe a group of disorders, including fibromyalgia, chronic fatigue syndrome, and irritable bowel syndrome, that share common features of MUS without clear medical pathology.

Grounding A technique used to bring awareness back to the body and the present moment, often through sensory experiences like feeling the ground beneath the feet. In TBMA, grounding helps individuals feel more stable and centred during emotional processing.

Health Anxiety (Hypochondriasis) Excessive worry or fear about having a serious medical condition, often despite reassurance from doctors. Individuals with MUS may also have health anxiety, leading to ongoing concerns about their unexplained symptoms.

Holistic This is characterised by the treatment of the whole person, taking into account mental and social factors, rather than just the symptoms of an illness.

Interoception The sense of the internal state of the body, including sensations like hunger, thirst, heartbeat or tension. TBMA uses interoceptive awareness to help individuals recognise how their emotions and thoughts manifest physically.

Learning Ecology A learning ecology as defined by Siemens (2007, p. 63) as "the space in which learning occurs". The characteristics of an ecology determine what can exist within it and learning ecologies are structured to serve a particular aim or purpose. It is used as a way of showing relationships between concepts.

Learned Helplessness This is when a person becomes dependent and over time becomes used to depending on others, losing agency.

Medically Unexplained Symptoms (MUS) Physical symptoms for which no clear or consistent medical cause can be identified, despite thorough medical investigation. These symptoms often include pain, fatigue or gastrointestinal issues.

Mind-Body Connection The relationship between the mind's influence on the body and the body's influence on the mind. TBMA emphasises the reciprocal nature of this connection to foster greater emotional, mental and physical well-being with the focus on the body first and foremost as this is always the starting point.

Mindfulness A state of intentional focused attention on the present moment, acknowledging thoughts, feelings and bodily sensations without judgment. Mindfulness practices are integral to TBMA, encouraging participants to stay present and observe their inner experiences.

Movement Movements used intentionally within TBMA to facilitate emotional release, self-expression. These movements are often simple and accessible, focusing on enhancing the connection between mind and body.

Nonverbal Communication The expression of thoughts, feelings or states of being through body language, gestures, posture and movement, rather than spoken words. TBMA often focuses on interpreting and working with these forms of communication.

Participant This refers to the person taking part in a TBMA programme.

Phenomenological A type of research that seeks to explain the nature of things through the way people experience them. It translates literally as the "study of phenomena". In other words, it's the study of the meaning these things (or phenomena) have in the minds of the audience you're studying.

Psychoeducation   The process of educating individuals about the psychological and emotional aspects of their experiences. TBMA incorporates psychoeducation to help participants understand the connection between their physical sensations and emotional states.

Psychophysiological Response   The interaction between psychological factors and the body's physical responses. In MUS, stress, anxiety and emotions can trigger or exacerbate physical symptoms through psychophysiological mechanisms.

Psychosocial Stressors   Life events or ongoing stress that impact psychological and social well-being, potentially contributing to the development or exacerbation of MUS. Addressing these stressors is a key part of managing MUS.

Psychosomatic   Relating to the interaction between mind and body, where emotional or psychological factors contribute to physical symptoms. Although not employed as a term in the UK, bodily symptoms which are medically unexplained are often considered psychosomatic in nature, as emotional distress can manifest physically.

Resilience   The capacity to recover and adapt in the face of challenges or adversity. TBMA aims to enhance resilience by helping individuals develop stronger emotional and physical self-awareness and coping strategies.

Self-Compassion   Treating oneself with kindness and understanding, especially in moments of difficulty or emotional pain. TBMA promotes self-compassion by encouraging participants to accept and nurture both their physical and emotional experiences.

Self-Management   The ability to self-care, and the management of, or by, oneself, taking responsibility for one's own behaviour and wellbeing.

Self-Regulation   The ability to manage and control one's emotions, thoughts and physical reactions. TBMA supports the development of self-regulation skills through somatic and mindfulness practices, which help individuals handle stress or emotional triggers.

Somatic Awareness   The ability to be consciously aware of the sensations and experiences in the body. Somatic awareness is central to TBMA as it encourages individuals to connect with their physical sensations to better understand emotional or psychological issues.

Somatisation   The process by which psychological distress manifests as physical symptoms. However, in TBMA somatisation also includes the distress experienced by individuals suffering a known, medical bodily symptom.

Stress   A form of psychological pain. A state of worry or mental tension caused by a difficult situation. Stress is a natural human response that prompts us to address challenges and threats in our lives. Everyone experiences stress to some degree.

Somatoform Disorders   A group of psychiatric disorders in which patients experience physical symptoms that are inconsistent with or cannot be fully explained by medical conditions. This term has been removed from the DSM5.

Symptom   A symptom is a manifestation of disease apparent to the patient, while a sign is a manifestation of disease that the physician perceives. The sign is objective evidence, a symptom, subjective. Symptoms represent the complaints of the patient, and if severe, they drive the patient to the doctor.

Trauma-Informed   An approach to care that recognises the impact of trauma on an individual's body, mind and emotions. TBMA is often trauma-informed, meaning it is sensitive to the needs of individuals who have experienced trauma and provides a safe, supportive space for healing.

This glossary covers important terms emphasising the complex interaction of mind, body and emotional states in the presentation of medically unexplained and explained symptoms as related to TBMA.

Reference

Siemens, G. (2007). Connectivism: Creating a learning ecology in distributed environments. In T. Hug (Ed.), *Didactics of Microlearning: Concepts, Discourses and Examples* (pp. 53–68). Waxmann Verlag.

Author and Subject Index

Note: Pages in *italics* refer to figures, pages in bold refer to tables.

For Product Safety Concerns and Information please contact our EU
representative GPSR@taylorandfrancis.com
Taylor & Francis Verlag GmbH, Kaufingerstraße 24, 80331 München, Germany